Nursing and Humanities

The humanities have long been recognized as having a place in nursing knowledge, and have been used in education, theory, and research by nurses. However, the place of humanities in nursing has always remained ambiguous. This book offers an in-depth exploration of the relationship between humanities and nursing.

The book starts with a survey of the history of humanities in nursing, in comparison with medical humanities and in the context of interdisciplinary health humanities. There is a description of applications of humanities within nursing. A central section offers an argument for placing the humanities firmly within a mixed model of nursing knowledge that is based upon embodied cognition. Further chapters explore these ideas through a series of essays on topics looking at nursing using viewpoints from the humanities. The concluding chapter considers present and future trends in nursing and the continuing need for humanities voices in developing nursing knowledge.

Nursing and Humanities is intended primarily for nurse academics and graduate students, who have an interest in nursing theory, applications of arts and humanities in education, and qualitative research approaches. It will also interest practicing nurses who are looking for an account of nursing that combines the technical and the human.

Graham McCaffrey is Associate Professor in the Faculty of Nursing, University of Calgary, Canada. He is Assistant Editor for the *Journal of Applied Hermeneutics*.

Routledge Research in Nursing and Midwifery

For more information about this series, please visit: www.routledge.com/
Routledge-Research-in-Nursing/book-series/RRIN

Nursing and Humanities

Graham McCaffrey

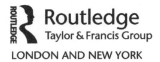

Routledge
Taylor & Francis Group

LONDON AND NEW YORK

First published 2020
by Routledge
4 Park Square, Milton Park, Abingdon, Oxon OX14 4RN
605 Third Avenue, New York, NY 10017

First issued in paperback 2023

Routledge is an imprint of the Taylor & Francis Group, an informa business

British Library Cataloguing-in-Publication Data
A catalogue record for this book is available from the British Library

Library of Congress Cataloging-in-Publication Data
Names: McCaffrey, Graham, author.
Title: Nursing and humanities/Graham McCaffrey.
Description: Milton Park, Abingdon, Oxon ; New York, NY : Routledge,
2020. | Includes bibliographical references and index.
Identifiers: LCCN 2019051087 (print) | LCCN 2019051088 (ebook) |
ISBN 9780367347765 (hardback) | ISBN 9780429327889 (ebook)
Subjects: LCSH: Nursing–Philosophy. | Medicine and the humanities.
Classification: LCC RT84.5 .M3785 2020 (print) | LCC RT84.5 (ebook) |
DDC 610.7301–dc23
LC record available at https://lccn.loc.gov/2019051087
LC ebook record available at https://lccn.loc.gov/2019051088

ISBN: 978-1-03-257086-0 (pbk)
ISBN: 978-0-367-34776-5 (hbk)
ISBN: 978-0-429-32788-9 (ebk)

DOI: 10.4324/9780429327889

Publisher's Note
The publisher has gone to great lengths to ensure the quality of this reprint but
points out that some imperfections in the original copies may be apparent.

Contents

Acknowledgements

My idea for this book has had a long evolution and I have many people to thank who have helped me to shape my thinking about humanities and nursing. Early in my graduate education, Dr. Nancy Moules introduced me – as she has so many students – to the possibilities of hermeneutic philosophy for exploring sensitive questions of human relating at the heart of nursing. I thank her too for reading a draft of the book. My doctoral supervisor, Dr. Shelley Raffin-Bouchal gave me unstinting support for my pursuit of the unlikely-seeming question of what Buddhist thought might have to say about mental health nursing. I have had many stimulating conversations interlaced with themes from the book with my colleague Dr. Lorraine Venturato. Not long after joining the Faculty of Nursing at the University of Calgary, I ran into Melanie Boyd, a university librarian whom I knew from a local Zen group – our conversation that day and subsequent work together brought humanities and health to the centre of my attention. I have had the good fortune to work with Dr. Tom Rosenal, a generous and determined advocate for the humanities in health care based at the Cumming School of Medicine in Calgary. Much of the orientation for the first part of the book comes out of subsequent work with Tom and other members of the Health Humanities group. And deep thanks to my wife Amanda Barber who kept me grounded and encouraged me through long days of writing.

Introduction

In the province of Alberta, Canada, where I am a Registered Nurse (RN), our statutory licensing body has a document laying out the competencies required in RNs entering practice. One of its stipulations is that the new nurse, "Incorporates knowledge from nursing science, social sciences, *humanities*, and health-related research into plans of care" [italics added] (College and Association of Registered Nurses of Alberta, 2019, p. 6). What does this mean? Why should registered nurses incorporate knowledge from the humanities into their plans of care, and what knowledge is this exactly, and how are they supposed to apply it? I am heartened but a little puzzled by the inclusion of humanities in this list. It shows they are important for nurses, but there is nothing in the rest of the document that makes clear *why* they are important. In this book, I endeavour to work out some answers to that question and to understand how it is that the humanities can be visible and yet obscure at the same time, in a document that lays out, point by point, the requirements of a nurse entering into fully licensed, professionally responsible practice for the first time.

Through researching and writing this book, I have come to think in terms of the relationship between nursing and the humanities. This book is about that relationship. By thinking in terms of a relationship, there is room to look at its trajectory over time, finding aspects of continuity and change, and at its many different aspects. It makes it possible to see more clearly why the humanities have always been present in nursing, yet often half hidden among categories like caring or qualitative research. Other concerns have often taken priority over a clear delineation of what practices and knowledge from the humanities can bring to nursing. My account is only one telling of the relationship, among many possibilities. I have dug deep into the nursing literature to anchor my version in what has gone before, and to connect it to current developments in the emergent field of health humanities. Nevertheless, as the book progresses, I have framed nursing and humanities following some of my own interests and concerns to ground humanities within a complex discipline that always comes down to embodied human experience, and which is fundamentally reliant on scientific knowledge and technical expertise. For some readers, I will have missed out something important, made the wrong connection, and either under- or over-emphasized some aspect of the relationship. I can only take responsibility for the trails I have chosen to pursue and say I have done my best to show how and why I have taken them. I have tried to establish the vital importance of the humanities for nursing and to show that plurality and diversity are intrinsic to what makes them important.

Meaning-making and metaphor

The relationship between humanities and nursing has deep roots. Both are broad areas of human activity that stem from basic social impulses. Underlying the humanities, meaning-making is an inescapable part of human life. It is only through finding meaning in things that we arrive at values and purposes, which are meanings in juxtaposition with other meanings. Meanings are fuelled by emotions, by the levels of intensity we give our likes and dislikes, attractions and repulsions. We strive over and over to express meaning, in language, images, shapes, sounds, and bodily movements. Language has us, making metaphors even out of our most basic orientation to the world as Lakoff and Johnson (2003) have shown. Human meaning-making is the business of the arts and humanities; in the unending urge to expression through art forms of all kinds, through digging deep into what it means to be human in philosophy and religion, or mapping meanings across time in historical writing and research. Individual meanings, from those things that matter to us moment to moment, which may be trivial in themselves, to the momentous events in each person's life, are always connected by root systems of interlinked meanings into shared cultural eco-systems. Arts and humanities carry fibrous connections of the complex social life of human beings.

Nursing standpoint

Into this picture, nursing enters with its own standpoint, its own concerns, values, and histories. In personifying nursing, I do not mean to elide the vast variety of what nurses do around the world, let alone the diversity of individuals who have taken up nursing as an occupation. But nursing represents a bandwidth of human activity that moves along common vectors of morality and purpose, that manifests in response to health and illness, that takes shape within structures of institutions and knowledge through which health care is provided. Everything about such a high-level definition invites questions – whose institutions, which knowledge, whose idea of health? Humanities give us the means to explore deeply into how nursing and nurses affect and are affected by our common human life. It may be questions of empathy and compassion, in momentary encounters that can relieve suffering or sometimes aggravate it; or of political structures in which nurses are caught up, leading to decisions about who gets what care that nurses are expected to enact; or even of excellence in carrying out a technical procedure, using what the philosopher Richard Kearney has noted is the tact in contact, since "to learn to touch well is to learn to live well, that is, *tactfully*" (Kearney, 2015, p. 20).

Nursing, like the humanities, is centred on human experience and human communication. Nursing moreover is about certain kinds of experience and communication, circulating through questions of health, that are directed at defined goals. As such, it entails much more than the humanities by themselves can provide. And yet, there is a core of trained attention on the experience of the suffering other that calls for the descriptive, sensory, interpretive, critical, questioning capacities of the humanities to keep nursing grounded in the endlessly rich worlds of human lives in which nurses do their work.

Overview of chapters

The book falls into three parts. The first two chapters are about the history of the relationship between nursing and humanities. For several years I have been involved in an interdisciplinary group that promotes Health Humanities at the University of Calgary. I have often been asked by medical colleagues, schooled in medical humanities, to describe the place of humanities in nursing. The question has always partly baffled me, not because I had nothing to report, but because it was hard to know where to start, how to capture a diffuse array of interests and activities that pervades nursing education, research, and practice but which has never been gathered together under one roof, like medical humanities. Chapter 1 is my attempt at an answer, looking at how and why medical humanities came to be, in contrast with how and why nursing took a different route in its embrace of humanities. Starting out by comparing nursing to medicine is grounded in historical reality, but it is not prescriptive. Only by understanding how we got here can we make thoughtful choices about where to go next.

While I argue that it is important to understand past developments in medical humanities in comparison to nursing, I believe the future lies with the emerging, interdisciplinary world of health humanities. Here nursing has its own voice, coming with its own values, scope, and history. In trying to capture that voice, my hope is that nurses are encouraged to contribute all the more to developments in the wider movement of health humanities. In Chapter 2, I review the many ways in which nurses have taken up the humanities without the umbrella of a defined movement of nursing humanities. This chapter gives some of the how-to of using humanities in nursing education and research, drawing on a wide and disparate nursing literature. One chapter is not enough to cover the whole range of applications that nurses have found for the humanities so I include landmark sources and highlight areas of education, history, and philosophy. The chapter concludes with a discussion of humanities in relation to the much debated "art of nursing".

Chapters 3 to 5 are theoretical, exploring ideas about the nature of nursing and how the humanities fit into a variegated picture of nursing. Chapter 3 revisits the perennial question of what nursing is, and I suggest a naturalized view of nursing grounded in prosocial human drives that are nonetheless always culturally inflected. I carry on the theme of culture to consider how nursing is always shaped and enacted by institutions. From these influences, I arrive at a qualified view of humanism as a type of practice. Chapter 4 is about the art and science of nursing, and takes the syncretic view that that nursing must include both. It is not a question of which matters more, or which is most essential, but pragmatically of what demands they each make and how they emerge through actual nursing practice. Whereas in much of nursing theory, the art and science of nursing have been put into opposition, or at best uneasy cohabitation, I argue for a materially grounded view of nursing as human activity that is consistent with both scientific explanation and cultural meaning-making. I introduce three thinkers who have advanced mixed ways of thinking, highlighting the role of interpretation for nursing. In Chapter 5 I look at developments in embodied cognition that I see as a good fit with the multivalence of nursing and that reemphasize the centrality of human-to-human contact in nursing. Embodied cognition is not new to nursing theory, but I offer a new synthesis by emphasizing the humanities in a picture of nursing that follows the affective, embodied, and encultured ramifications of embodied cognition. Chapters 3, 4, and 5 together have an arc of a new, integrative account of nursing that puts the humanities into the mix with the sciences and the materiality of practice.

Chapters 6, 7, and 8 are separate essays on themes about nursing, thinking with the humanities, based upon earlier pieces of work. Chapter 6 takes up the concept of the *pharmakon*, a substance with ambivalent effects of healing and/or poisoning, and puts health humanities into the place of such a substance. I use its ambivalence to question comfortable assumptions about compassion in nursing, and to consider the role of necessity in forming care. Chapter 7 is about prose and poetry in nursing. I look at how different literary forms can do different things to show or make sense of aspects of nursing. I discuss narratives from a variety of angles and then contrast how lyric poetry can powerfully illuminate moments of intense experience. Chapter 8 draws on work from my doctoral dissertation, where I took concepts from Buddhist thought and applied them to problematic areas in the practice of mental health nurses on acute hospital units. I take up the thread of interconnection in Buddhist thought and consider how it might help in articulating the many aspects of interrelationship that occur in nursing.

Chapter 9 turns attention towards the future of nursing and humanities. It is not prophecy, though I discuss some futurist projections, taking them as mirrors to trends that are already at work. With various conceptions of what it means to be post-human roaming the landscape, I reassert the continuing importance of the humanities to focus on the human in nursing, as it is affected by advances in technology and health science. Humanities give us ways to track the shifting borderlines between human and non-human shift.

Who the book is for

Humanities turn up in nursing in education, research, theory, and practice. Even if not named as such, they are there when students look at a film or novel to gain insight into patient experience, or when qualitative researchers try to get close to experience and understand it in new ways. They are present when nurses need to bridge cultural difference to effect good care. The humanities have wide relevance to nursing and yet I suspect there are relatively few nurses either in practice or in academia who consciously think about the role of humanities in their own practice. This book is intended as a contribution to the tradition of writing about the humanities in nursing and is primarily aimed at nurses working in education and research who are already tuned in to that tradition. I have offered an integrative account of nursing, and although I am by no means the first to do so, I offer a new dimension in starting from the relationship between nursing and the humanities. Thus, the book will hopefully appeal to readers who are interested in nursing theory broadly. I hope too, that it will reach nurses in practice who are drawn to perennial, fuzzy questions of human relating that make nursing such demanding and rewarding work, and which no amount of data seems able to answer; nurses who turn to literature, poetry, art, music, and film to make connections between their own lives and the myriad forms of cultural expression that human beings use to find themselves in the world.

Note on usage. I have followed the example of the authors of the recent book *Health Humanities* (Crawford, Brown, Baker, Tischler, & Abrams, 2015, p. 12) in folding arts into the term humanities, rather than using the phrase "arts and humanities" each time. I have broken my own rule on occasion, when I wanted to emphasize the creation of artistic works under the wider category of the humanities.

References

College and Association of Registered Nurses of Alberta. (2019). *Entry-level competencies for the practice of registered nurses*. Edmonton, AB: Author.

Crawford, P., Brown, B., Baker, C., Tischler, V., & Abrams, B. (2015). *Health humanities*. Basingstoke, UK: Palgrave Macmillan.

Kearney, R. (2015). The wager of carnal hermeneutics. In R. Kearney & B. Treanor (Eds.), *Carnal hermeneutics* (pp. 15–56). New York, NY: Fordham University Press.

Lakoff, G., & Johnson, M. (2003). *Metaphors we live by*. Chicago, IL: The University of Chicago Press.

1 Nursing and the humanities

Medical and health humanities

In this chapter I give an overview of the current context for thinking about nursing and the humanities, in relation to the field of medical humanities and the trend towards interdisciplinary health humanities. I start with medical humanities because it is more well established and knowing something about this related field and its origins helps to clarify what is different for nursing in taking up the humanities. I then discuss the emerging field of health humanities and suggesting how nursing can contribute to an interdisciplinary field. In the final section, I introduce voices from the humanities themselves, expressing ideas about the value of the humanities and seeing how they meet up with perspectives that start out from healthcare.

Medical humanities

Medical humanities, as a term, is well established and well recognized in a way that nursing humanities is not. One reason is that medical humanities evolved out of developments in medical education during the late nineteenth century when modern professionalized nursing was only just coming into being. Medical education in the West has its roots in the humanist education of early modernity, when learning from the Classical world informed all branches of knowledge and humanism embraced both cultural and naturalist dimensions of human life. Following the development of scientific method starting in the seventeenth century, there began to be a divergence between the natural sciences and humanities. Medicine, then as now, was compelled to follow the undeniable successes of science as applied to knowledge of physiology, illness, and treatments, yet as a practical occupation it could not be wholly subsumed into the natural sciences.

Bleakley (2015) puts the first appearance of the term "medical humanities" in 1948 although Cole, Carlin, and Carson (2015) note that it did not come into common usage until the 1980s and 1990s. However, there was already a sense of dislocation or even identity crisis, at least among some physicians, in the face of rapid advances in scientific medicine in the latter half of the nineteenth century. Germ theory, anaesthesia and surgical procedures created new demands for the education of doctors as scientifically knowledgeable and technically skilled. The associated trend towards specialization was seen as a threat to the unified identity of the profession (Cole et al., 2015).

Advocates of restoring the moral core of medicine initially saw history as the best way of realigning the profession with its highest traditions. According to one historian of medicine, "history was to be the cornerstone of a new humanism in medicine that would promote cross-cultural dialogue between the sciences and the humanities" (Warner, 2011, p. 92). This initial turn towards the humanities was not made in opposition to the rise of modern scientific medicine, but as a corrective to its alienating tendencies. History was considered the most direct way of reconnecting with the humanist tradition of education, predicated on "an ideal of the 'gentleman-physician' well versed in the classic liberal arts" (Warner, 2011, p. 92). William Osler, a prominent doctor of this period, is the figure most associated with the concern for the humanity of medicine. As well as looking back to humanism, he was an advocate of reform in clinical teaching to emphasize bedside teaching and face-to-face patient contact (Bleakley, 2015). At the same time, there was an element of maintaining prestige and class status based on a traditional education in so-called high culture. The concern for humanism in medicine brought with it questions about quite what this meant, and how it was, or could be, linked to the humanities. Harvey Cushing, a neurosurgeon who like Osler was both an advocate of scientific progress and concerned with the loss of humanist values, worried that "the very terms humanism, humanities and humanization could be vague and their meanings fluid" (Warner, 2011, p. 93). This is a question that continues to show up in the field of medical humanities, and for that matter in health humanities or nursing humanities.

The next signal figure in trying to establish a place for the humanities in medical education is Abraham Flexner, who wrote a report on medical education for the Carnegie Foundation in 1910 which was massively influential (Doukas, McCullough, & Wear, 2010). Flexner advocated for higher and more uniform standards in medical education and saw the physician primarily as a scientist. However, he also assumed that applicants for medical school would come with a sound, broadly based education, and that the practice of medicine required contextualized judgement that was best achieved through a grounding in the humanities (Doukas et al., 2010).

Thus, alongside the emergence of modern medicine from the late nineteenth century onwards, there has been a concern with the potential for the loss of humanity, ethical clarity, and cohesive professional identity in the face of reductionism, standardization, and specialization. It is worth noting that these ideals do not all amount to the same thing. Professionalism can either denote (as it usually does in relation to medical humanities) a comportment of concern and respect towards individual patients, or a self-interested concern with group status. As Cushing noted early on, the handy etymological associations between humane-humanism-humanities can elide the differences between them and slide over more complex questions of what is meant by humanism, or if there is any good reason why the humanities would make people more humane. In addition to these questions, there are some characteristics of medical humanities that are already visible in these early developments that have shaped the field and are important to note when it comes to distinguishing the very different course of humanities in relation to nursing. First, medical humanities are closely associated with medical education. Medical humanities are one answer to the question of how to produce doctors who are not only competent but also kind. Second, medical humanities are involved over a concern with professionalism in the first sense above – questions of comportment and disposition towards others.

The questions raised by the early advocates of humanities in medicine, such as Osler, Cushing, and Flexner did not go away in the early decades of the twentieth century, but in the 1960s and 1970s there began to be a renewed attention to humanities. History of medicine, for example, was taken up less as a way of sustaining tradition and in a more critical, reflective way to examine medical culture (Warner, 2011). Edmund Pellegrino was a leading voice for humanizing medicine in the 1970s (Cole et al., 2015). He started from the assertion that medicine, though necessarily involving scientific knowledge and skills, was not reducible to science. "Medicine enjoys a unique position among disciplines – as a humane science whose technology must ever be person-oriented. Its practitioners are, therefore, under an extraordinary mandate to live and work within a humanistic frame" (Pellegrino, 1974, p. 1288). Here he is making a point that is not new or unique, but worth quoting because it states so well the relational and ethical commitments that are inherent in medical practice (though I question whether these are unique to medicine as Pellegrino states here, or applicable also to other health professions including nursing). From this standpoint, he asks, "What does it mean to educate a humanist physician in contemporary society?" (p. 1288). For Pellegrino, a grounding in the traditional canon of Western humanism is less important than a liberal education that serves to cultivate socially and contextually aware, other-oriented care. He is more interested ultimately in values that will humanize the physician's practice with scientific knowledge than in any particular attainment in arts or literature.

Medical humanities have developed in scope since the 1970s, becoming recognized as a distinctive field, as a widely accepted component of medical education, and as a focus for institutions and publications. In recent years, there has been a flurry of excellent new books in the field, including Cole, Carlin, and Carson's *Medical Humanities* textbook and Bleakley's *Medical Humanities and Medical Education*, both in 2015. I draw primarily on these two sources to give a brief survey of the range of goals for medical humanities that are currently motivating those working in the field.

Cole et al. (2015) identify four goals for medical humanities, as "bridge between science and experience" (p. 9), "educating more humane physicians" (p. 10), "recovering a learned profession" (p. 11), and "moral critique and political aspiration" (p. 11). Taking each of these in turn, bridging science and experience starts with the concrete clinical situation that the physician deals with objective data to diagnose and treat a disorder of some kind, while the patient has the experience of their own self altered by illness (and the physician too is an experiencing subject, however focused he or she is on rational evaluation of information).

Arts and literature have always been a means of conveying experience, of imaginative transport into other realms of experience that can then also be shared, discussed, and compared with others. Thus, the humanities can provide ways of gaining insight into the doubled experience of objective and subjective that is a mark of modern medicine, and as we have seen a preoccupation for at least some physicians since the advent of modern medicine.

Educating more humane physicians is probably the most prevalent goal for medical humanities, partly because it becomes visible in the complicated and politicized environment of curriculum and programme design in medical schools. Advocacy of medical humanities is concretized in competition for space in crowded schedules. It has been driven by a concern that empathy in medical students declines over the course of their studies (Neumann et al., 2011). Using resources from the arts and the humanities to prompt reflection and alternative perspective taking, to look at things from others' points of view, is intended to support empathy and compassion in clinical practice.

Recovering a learned profession is a goal that reaches back, through Pellegrino, to Osler and Flexner and the idea that practitioners with broad learning can bring richer understanding to their professional lives. It also reasserts a claim to the value of pursuing intellectual questions that do not have an immediate instrumental value or that cannot be answered with quantified measures.

The fourth goal, of humanities as moral critique and political aspirations, is a development of the critical self-awareness that became a feature of medical humanities, as well as many other disciplines, in the 1960s and 1970s. Technical advances in medicine have afforded effective, even life-saving treatments, but have raised unforeseen questions such as the prolongation of life with progressive conditions, iatrogenic side effects, or the fair distribution of expensive resources. None of these kinds of questions are answerable by the technologies themselves, nor by a simple resort to evidence which might be used to support opposing positions. History and philosophy provide ways of thinking about difficult moral and political problems, while arts and literature can be used to explore ambiguity, paradox, and indeed, the tragic.

For Bleakley, the "critical" (2015, p. 33) medical humanities are of foremost importance, serving the project of what he calls "the democratizing of medicine – shifting medical practice from an authority-led hierarchy that is doctor-centred to a patient-centred and interprofessional team process" (p. 2). He argues that "the humanities can offer an education into seeing otherwise" (p. 16). Seeing otherwise, being open and responsive to other perspectives, is not only a matter of empathy towards individuals, but a political commitment to reflect critically upon established values and institutions, and to exploring alternative ways of thinking and doing. He notes a tension between viewing the arts as a healing force, essentially as soothing and calming, and the intention of many artists to disrupt the status quo, to upset familiar assumptions that may in fact conceal problematic relationships. He envisages a pluralistic landscape of "interacting networks" (p. 32), at times in tension, and at times in productive conversation with each other, that draw on the humanities in different ways in pursuit of different goals.

Narrative medicine

One development in medical humanities that deserves separate mention is narrative medicine, since it has assumed a major place in the field (Charon, 2006; Frank, 2002, 2013; Kumagi, 2008). Narrative medicine pays attention to patient stories, to what the experience of illness, as opposed to the diagnosis of a disease or condition, means to the person undergoing it. Narrative medicine is rooted in the basic medical practice of taking a history, but is a reaction against a narrow focus on gathering information in order to make a diagnosis, which puts the priority on the needs of the physician rather than the actual concerns of the patient. It may also exclude or discount information that does turn out to have a bearing on how best the physician should proceed to heal the person, and not just treat the presenting problem. Narrative medicine restores the story to a medical history. One of the key works in the development of narrative medicine is by Arthur Kleinman (1988) who was both a psychiatrist and an anthropologist. He was alive to the importance of the patient's inner life and experience, as well as to how individual illness is expressed through a dense mesh of cultural values and meanings. More recently, Rita Charon has developed narrative medicine by bringing to bear the knowledge and methods of literary analysis to the doctor-patient dialogue. The doctor thus becomes not just a professional seeking prescribed pieces of information, but the audience for a narrative, an informed audience attuned to how meaning appears through plot, character, and purpose (Charon, 2006; Charon & Montello, 2002). Narrative medicine is important because it has become a major element in medical humanities and because it is a significant example of how interdisciplinary approaches can be brought to bear on clinical practice. Its wider significance, is that narrative is one opening – though not the only one – to the role of language and dialogue in clinical encounters, education, and research for all health professionals.

Nursing and humanities

Against the background of medical humanities, there is no such well-defined tradition in nursing, although there has been much debate in nursing literature about the humanities. Davis wrote an editorial in the *American Journal of Nursing* in 2003 calling for the systematic inclusion of humanities in nursing education along the lines of medical humanities, under the heading "Nursing humanities: The time has come" (p. 13). It is unusual, however, to find the term nursing humanities as a distinct category in nursing literature. It has never caught on in direct equivalence to medical humanities, although there has been no shortage of engagement with the humanities on the part of nurses, as clinicians, educators, scholars, and researchers.

Others who have promoted the humanities in nursing have sometimes taken medical humanities in a generic sense to include health professions more generally, such that they could be imported into nurse education (Corri, 2003; Robb & Murray, 1992). Darbyshire combined "medical/nursing humanities" (1994, p. 856) to describe a new course using arts and humanities within an interdisciplinary health studies programme. Dellasega et al. (2007) advanced a model for interdisciplinary education at the "humanities interface of nursing and medicine" (p. 174). Variations in terminology show an interest in medical humanities on the part of nurses and often a desire to find in the humanities a bridge between disciplines.

Authors have reflected on why nursing humanities have never developed as a discrete field like medical humanities. Dellasega et al. (2007) identified a move away from humanities in nursing curricula during the 1980s with increasing amounts of science content following developments in medical science, even while medical humanities had been becoming more prominent since the 1970s. Davis (2003) suggested that nurses tend to think that they are less in need than medical students of the humanizing influence promised by exposure to humanities.

There may be something in this when you compare the historical trajectories of the two professions. Warner, in his historical survey of medical humanities observed that, "… humanistic medicine first emerged at precisely the moment when modern Western biomedicine became ascendant" (Warner, 2011, p. 91). This was at the same historical moment that modern nursing emerged, with its vexed relationship with medicine right out of the gate. Nurses claimed to encompass precisely the humane values that doctors were felt to be shedding under the pressure of scientific medicine. Thus, nursing never experienced a rupture between an earlier perception of itself and a new, modern, scientific identity. Nurses took on as part of their professional identity caring for each person, and creating the best conditions for healing without feeling a need to find their way back to what Kleinman (1988) dubbed "illness narratives" by means of the humanities. Later on, in the latter part of the twentieth century, with the growth of academic nursing and theory and in the face of rapid technological change, there was still not much movement towards the humanities as such. Instead, theoreticians tended to double down on caring and holism as the distinguishing characteristics of nursing, packaged into elaborate theories. The need for grand theory was justified under the rubric of nursing science, despite the overtly metaphysical and spiritual content of some theories.

None of this means that the humanities have not always continued to play an important part in nursing but it is a suggested tracing of the absence of any close equivalent to medical humanities. When it comes to work by advocates of the humanities in nursing, a common theme is indeed that they have value as a complement and a corrective to the technical and scientific in nursing (Corri, 2003; Dellasega et al., 2007; Sullivan, 1996). The fact that nursing humanities has not developed as a discrete field of study and practice does not take away from the rich, productive relationship that exists between nursing and humanities. There are advantages to having a recognizable field like medical humanities, which lends coherence and identity to projects in education or research, or to pro-grammes and academic positions. It is important, however, not to lose sight of the position the humanities have in nursing, overlapping with some of the ethical, professional, and interpersonal concerns they are expected to address in medicine. In nursing, we have tended not to think about patient narratives, or concern for the patient's contextual experience of illness, as a special job for the humanities but as a normal part of the scope of nursing. Looking at nursing through the lens of the humanities, however, can give us fresh perspectives on things that are already deeply familiar, and suggest new avenues in education and research.

Medical humanities/health humanities

In line with a wider trend towards interprofessional collaboration in health care services, the field of medical humanities has shifted towards a more interdisci-plinary approach. (I am making a distinction between inter*professional* collabo-ration between health care professions in clinical settings, and inter*disciplinary* collaborations that may cross the boundary between academic and clinical worlds, and can also include non-health care disciplines from the arts and humanities.) Even those authors who have chosen to stick to the term medical humanities have felt the need to explain their choice. Bleakley (2015), for example, argues that either medical humanities are aligned with medical educa-tion in which case the designation is simply descriptive, or that potential collab-orators "will meet healthcare in general even as they work with doctors" (p. 44) who are members of multiprofessional teams. This seems to be another way of saying that "medical" is a good enough blanket term for what goes on in health care, though for those of us in other professions it can feel like a continuation of a long-established hegemony. Bleakley makes a further point that the term health lends itself to a kind of complacency of well-being that blunts the critical value of the arts, and endorses a conservative "homeostasis model of medicine" (p. 26). This introduces a valid concern about the valences of the word health in modern discourses of "health and wellness" or of individuals "taking responsib-ility for their own health", but these complications hardly seem any more of a reason to avoid the term than does the historic baggage of the medical.

Cole et al. (2015) also address the question, acknowledging that "medical humanities" can be seen as expressing a traditional hierarchy of medicine over other health care professions. They express support for the "spirit of inclusivity and equality" (p. 7) sought for in the emergence of health humanities but explain their decision to stick with medical humanities on the pragmatic grounds that (a) most of the scholarship on the area is focused on medicine and (b) the scope of their book is medical. Both of the above discussions make ref-erence to Jones, Wear, and Friedman's (2014) *Health Humanities Reader*, whose authors opted for the more inclusive term. In their introduction to the edited collection, they outline the background of the medical humanities and argue it is time "to adopt the more encompassing, contemporary, and accurate label of the current academic enterprise – the *health humanities*" (p. 6). Interestingly, out of 58 contributors listed in the volume, 35 are listed as either MD or having an appointment at a medical school, and most of the rest are either humanities scholars or have appointments in health sciences' departments with no specific discipline mentioned. I could find only one contributor who was identified as a nurse. This suggests there is some truth in Cole et al.'s defence of medical humanities, that this is how things are, but the fact that terminology is being debated is itself sign of a shift. Jones et al. state their intent to position their work as an argument and agent for changing the balance.

The most thoroughgoing advocacy for health humanities to date is in Crawford et al.'s (2015) book of the same title. Paul Crawford, the lead author, is Professor of Health Humanities at the University of Nottingham in the UK. The authors make a powerful case for a broad, inclusive vision of health humanities that takes account of changes in health care, of the involvement of non-professional groups as well as unpaid caregivers in care, and of traditions of therapeutic applications of arts and humanities. While looking towards the development of an inclusive field of health humanities, they note the different disciplinary horizons that bring a variety of perspectives to bear on the interface between humanities and health. Pluralism within a sense of shared community can bring different, even conflicting, assumptions into engagement with each other. The authors of *Health Humanities* make clear that while they are interested in the therapeutic possibilities of the humanities, they are no less emphatic about bringing critical theories to bear on established beliefs, structures, and practices.

Nursing humanities/health humanities

The relationship between humanities and nursing discussed above, though less strictly defined and organized than medical humanities, puts nurses who are committed to developing humanities in nursing in a good position from which to contribute to the health humanities. Having less of an established structure to reconfigure to the emergent interdisciplinary approach, nurses ought to be adaptable to different forms of interchange and collaboration. Nursing, nonetheless, has a distinctive voice, as does each discipline, with its own goals, values, and histories.

Standpoint epistemology is a way of trying to delineate the distinctiveness of the nursing perspective and thus to describe the relationship with the humanities more fully. I am taking up the concept of nursing standpoint from the 2010 book about nursing knowledge by the philosopher Mark Risjord, but whereas his objective is to situate nursing knowledge within a flexible conception of science, I am suggesting that there is a nursing standpoint that will influence how nurses make use of the humanities.

Risjord (2010), who explains that he borrowed standpoint epistemology from feminism, argues that nursing meets four criteria for having a standpoint from which its knowledge base can be defined. All four connect with the socio-political position of nursing in relation to medicine: first, that the nurse in health care is in a position of less power, second that nursing activity is largely determined by the priorities of doctors, third that as a consequence, nursing work becomes invisible – essential but taken for granted – and fourth that nurses as a result have a doubled perspective of being comfortable both with medical ways of thinking and talking, and with a keener awareness of patients' experience, needs, and forms of expression. For Risjord, the significance of the nursing standpoint is that "moral or political values can be constitutive to scientific inquiry" (Risjord, 2010, p. 73).

While the situation of nurses in relation to medicine is a formative part of any nursing standpoint, it can be restrictive to think about nursing primarily in a subordinate position, or to focus on the nurse's place in health care without noting the power that nurses, by dint of their institutional authority, have over patients. Building upon the idea of the standpoint, I would add two further considerations. One is to think of the standpoint in relation to the horizon of concern. Horizon is a metaphor that the hermeneutic philosopher Gadamer (1960/2004) uses in his work to point out the limits of knowledge and the changeability of knowledge, since what is visible, or out of sight beyond the horizon changes as we move ourselves. Our standpoint therefore, as Risjord argues, helps to define what we are able to see and directs us towards what we expect to see, but if it is moveable and not fixed then familiar sights can disappear and new, unexpected objects come into view. I am not suggesting nurses can simply drop their standpoint at will and choose another one but that, for example, within nursing the multiplicity of clinical specialties and workplaces does give rise to variations in style and emphasis. Over the years, some nursing colleagues when finding out I worked in mental health have said something like, "I could never work in mental health – it takes a certain kind of person!" – well, maybe, but I can say the same to intensive care or paediatric nurses. There is a creative tension between what we share, in a basic orientation towards patients, or in working out collaborative relationships across professions, and what is different in our uses of technology or foregrounded knowledge, for example, of mental health assessment rather than pathophysiology. One of the pleasures for me of teaching an introductory course in nursing philosophy to new graduate students is hearing them compare experiences from diverse clinical areas, finding both their differences and commonalities.

Continuing this line of thinking, the second consideration is to elaborate on the standpoint from within nursing before looking at it in relation to other professions. A number of nursing theorists have proposed pluralist and integrative accounts of nursing. The Developmental Health Framework (Gottlieb & Gottlieb, 2007), for example, sets out the basis of nursing knowledge, grounded in biological and developmental science, but also incorporating human capacities to interpret their own situation, and to make decisions about how to cope in the face of change. Although rooted in naturalism, the framework takes account of subjective experience, social relationships, and cultural influences as part of the nursing engagement with others directed towards optimized, healthy coping. A very different approach, though sharing a similar concern with how to capture the complexity of nursing, is relational inquiry (Hartrick Doane & Varcoe, 2015) which makes relational interconnectedness the mobilizing concept for nursing. Relational inquiry is derived from the multi-layered actuality of nursing practice and the authors use it to examine how nurses are required to have a firm base of knowledge and sophisticated analytical skills and judgement if they are to take account of all the salient points of any situation and to practice with wide, alert peripheral vision.

Both frameworks are good examples of how nurses-thinking-about-nursing have moved on from grand theory design to more practical endeavours to reflect and articulate the complex challenges of practice. Neither of these theoretical accounts is about the humanities in nursing, or even mentions them directly, but they are helpful in pointing towards a nursing standpoint that includes the humanities within its horizon. They reflect the difficulty of bringing all the dimensions of nursing into a coherent whole and suggest that there is no final way of doing so, either. Representation of complexity is one of the arguments for turning to the humanities in health care, and nursing itself has its own complexity which demands more than one form of understanding.

Both frameworks, to varying degrees, include culture as one of the forces at play in nursing practice. Culture can be taken to mean different things. Within health care, it can refer to differences between professions, institutional social environments, or the atmosphere in a specific workplace; more broadly, it has the anthropological meaning of the whole of the traditions, values, technologies, arts, language of a given human group, or it can point to forms of human expression of meaning and value. Culture can be regarded through the social sciences as an object of study. There are times when that is the most useful vector of inquiry for nurses to produce knowledge about how the profession can best meet the health needs of society, and to understand the forces and structures that enable or inhibit them in doing so. Culture however, in every sense, is manifested through being lived out, and in doing so it often eludes easy categorization. Each of us partakes of different kinds of cultures, which make different kinds of demands of us, whether we are with family, in the workplace, or part of a group held together by custom, belief, and common purpose. Although there are identifiable forces that determine a nursing standpoint, it is also a space that permits movement, according to who adopts it and in relation to shifting horizons. The humanities are disciplines of close attention to cultural formation, expression, dissonance, and change.

Another way to think about how nursing can offer a distinctive contribution within the wider world of health humanities is through the philosopher Charles Taylor's (2007) concept of social imaginary. He employs this term to go beyond sociological categories, to capture how people "imagine their social existence, how they fit together with others, how things go on between them and their fellows, the expectations which are normally met, and the deeper normative notions and images which underlie these expectations" (p. 171). Social imaginaries are more than the sum of their parts, so that they include symbolic, ritual, and moral understandings that inform a coherent sense of a social group. In the UK for example, following the exposure of appalling and systematic neglect of patients at the Mid Staffordshire Hospital Trust and subsequent Francis Report (2013) into what happened, there was widespread complaint in the media that nurses had lost their compassion. Part of the problem according to some commentators was that there was no Matron to maintain standards. The figure of the Matron, historically a senior figure in nursing hierarchies in hospital, was transmogrified in the social imaginary into a stern, disciplined, yet ultimately caring figure who will make everything all right, like a mother comforting a frightened child in the middle of the night. Social imaginary is a useful way to explain the odd mixture of factual reporting, moral judgement, wishful thinking, and ignorance of modern nursing that went into the nostalgic demand for Matron. Gordon and Nelson (2006) have argued against what they call "the virtue script" (p. 13) in nursing, which presents an idealized view of nurses as caring, morally pure women and in doing so obscures the reality of their extensive knowledge and technical expertise. They have, in Taylor's terms, shed light on a social imaginary that exerts a powerful pull on nurses themselves as well as non-nurses. With its play of symbolic imagination and emotional appeal, the social imaginary of nursing can be rethought and reimagined through both the analytic humanities disciplines of history, philosophy, and literary criticism, as well as through artistic representation in literature, drama, or visual images.

Social imaginaries, according to Taylor, have a deep background such that, "sense-giving draws on our whole world, that is, our sense of our whole predicament in time and space, among others and in history" (p. 174). There is something shared in the social imaginary of nursing, as the Matron example demonstrates – nurses have a responsibility to articulate what they do, but they cannot be in full control of how others will see them. More positively, the shared background invites participation with other disciplines and professions in the health humanities, against the wider background of health care.

Crawford et al. (2015) in making their case for an interdisciplinary field of health humanities, say that, "despite vigorous debate and the conflicting assumptions of different disciplines … there is nevertheless a sense of community between contributors to the humanities in healthcare" (p. 13). This neatly captures the mixture of commonality and difference that exists among health care disciplines, which is in itself fertile ground for work using the humanities. Among the purposes Crawford et al. set out for health humanities is "to provide insight into the human condition" (p. 18), and health care as one venue for human life presents plenty of opportunities to explore and reflect upon how difference can be both challenging and stimulating, destructive or creative.

The humanities

If there is a need to work out the value of humanities for nursing and other health professions, scholars in the humanities have felt a need to justify the study of humanities itself. It is ironic that there is a revitalization of interest in the humanities in healthcare when there is anxiety within the humanities themselves about falling enrolments in humanities subjects in universities and cuts to programmes. A recent article in The New York Review of Books asked, "are the humanities history?" (Massing, 2019). Two recent works, from the US and UK respectively, give a sense of the arguments that have been marshalled to promote the study of the humanities that set out common ground with advocates in healthcare.

Martha Nussbaum, in her 2010 book *Not for Profit* makes a wholehearted case for the humanities being central to successful democratic societies. Nussbaum has a developmental argument for finding ways to educate people for compassion. She sees disgust as a fundamental part of early human development, by which a person learns to distinguish clean from dirty, and at higher levels of abstraction, desirable from undesirable. This is a necessary self-protective mechanism to inform judgements as people go about in the world, but is liable to bending towards attitudes of stigmatization and discrimination against people who are different to oneself and one's own group. Another fundamental aspect of human functioning, however, is the capacity for compassion and for seeing others in their own individuality, with their own outlook. For Nussbaum, these two forces compete within all of us. It is not that discrimination will be educated out of us with the right amount of humanities content, or that compassion is not dependent on circumstances. But she argues that an education in the humanities, with a goal of promoting good citizenship, has the resources to develop a disposition towards seeing things from others' points of view, of concern for others, and learning accurately about other groups in order to reduce thoughtless responses.

Some of the specific skills Nussbaum finds in the humanities are Socratic questioning, forming rational arguments, and being able to work out one's own opinions without deferring to dominant ideas. Humanities offer training, amongst other things, in assessing and synthesizing historical evidence, evaluating accounts of social justice, and appreciating the complexities of world religions. In the nexus of health care systems, someone with a disposition informed by such ways of thinking would be well placed to work sensitively with the values and meanings that patients and families bring with them into encounters with nurses.

Nussbaum further puts value on "the narrative imagination" (2010, p. 96) to be able to have some understanding of other people's feelings, ideas, and situations – not to claim to know other people from inside out, but to be able to comprehend their story well enough to shape goals of care that are both clinically sound and meaningful to the patient in terms of their own goals. Given her view that humans have competing drives towards affiliation and inclusion, or exclusion and dehumanization, she is not naïve enough to think that exposure to the humanities by itself is enough to strengthen the former, without being linked to an ethical vision of human dignity.

Helen Small, in her book *The Value of the Humanities* (2013), takes a less forthright approach and focuses more on the work of professional scholars in the humanities than on their role in the educational system as a whole (as she notes, Nussbaum's perspective draws on the American liberal arts tradition as opposed to the UK model of disciplinary specialization beginning in secondary education).

Small argues that any defence of the humanities must be pluralist, that any one purpose is not sufficient by itself. She works through five broad claims, including a more qualified version of Nussbaum's central argument that humanities can contribute to a well-functioning democratic politics, through practices of reflection and reasoned argument. Perhaps the most relevant of her claims from the standpoint of nursing and humanities is a close examination of the disciplinary distinctiveness of the humanities. Her, deliberately broad, definition of the humanities is the, "study of meaning-making practices of the culture, focusing on interpretation and evaluation with an indispensable element of subjectivity" (2013, p. 4). This goes to what it is that health professions require from the humanities alongside, but in addition to, scientific knowledge and algorithms. Where Small elaborates on the distinctive qualities of humanities compared to sciences, many of her points occur also in disciplinary debates about the value of qualitative research in nursing. She notes the humanities value qualitative over quantitative knowledge, interpretive over positivist thinking, individual experience, and the viewpoint of the perceiver in knowledge claims (2013, pp. 29–30).

Her other three areas of finding value for the humanities are in demonstrable economic value, the contribution to personal and social happiness, and valuing them for their own sake. I will not discuss them here, because they seem to me less immediately relevant to nursing. One point of relevance that does emerge, however, from seeing these arguments from humanities scholars is that for them, certain forms of health humanities would count among the instrumental uses of humanities. Within higher education, one thing we may have to offer in interdisciplinary collaborations are avenues for demonstrating practical applications of the humanities, and putting to the test some of the claims made for them.

Conclusion

The humanities are a crucial meeting ground for human cultural expression, reflection, and self-understanding. It is no wonder that people in healthcare professions, who are constantly exposed to others, often at times of extreme physical and emotional experiences, have turned to the arts and humanities to try to make sense of their world, to seek comfort or to become more critical, for healing or for questioning, or to ask questions that may never have good answers, but go on being asked. We are in a time of increasing emphasis in healthcare on interprofessional practice and education. Humanities, that appeal to human predicaments over and above disciplinary differences, are one way of establishing common ground, yet also of carefully holding and making use of the array of voices within healthcare.

References

Bleakley, A. (2015). *Medical humanities and medical education*. New York, NY: Routledge.

Charon, R. (2006). *Narrative medicine: Honoring the stories of illness*. New York, NY: Oxford University Press.

Charon, R., & Montello, M. (Eds.). (2002). *Stories matter: The role of narrative in medical ethics*. New York, NY: Routledge.

Cole, T.R., Carlin, N.S., & Carson, R.A. (2015). *Medical humanities*. New York, NY: Cambridge University Press.

Corri, C. (2003). Medical humanities in nurse education. *Nursing Standard, 17*(33), 38–40.

Crawford, P., Brown, B., Baker, C., Tischler, V., & Abrams, B. (2015). *Health humanities*. Basingstoke, UK: Palgrave Macmillan.

Darbyshire, P. (1994). Understanding caring through arts and humanities: A medical/nursing humanities approach to promoting alternative experiences of thinking and learning. *Journal of Advanced Nursing, 19*, 856–863.

Davis, C. (2003). Nursing humanities: The time has come. *American Journal of Nursing, 103*(2), 13.

Dellasega, C., Milone-Nuzzo, P., Curci, K.M., Ballard, J.O., & Kirch, D.G. (2007). The humanities interface of nursing and medicine. *Journal of Professional Nursing, 23*(3), 174–179.

Doukas, D.J., McCullough, L.B., & Wear, S. (2010). Reforming medical education in ethics and humanities by finding common ground with Abraham Flexner. *Academic Medicine, 85*(2), 318–322.

Francis, R. (2013). *Report of the Mid Staffordshire NHS Foundation Trust public inquiry*. London, UK: The Stationery Office.

Frank, A.W. (2002). *At the will of the body: Reflections on illness*. New York, NY: Mariner.

Frank, A.W. (2013). *The wounded storyteller: Body, illness and ethics* (2nd ed.). Chicago, IL: University of Chicago Press.

Gadamer, H.G. (1960/2004). *Truth and method*. (J. Weinsheimer & D.G. Marshall, Trans.). New York, NY: Continuum.

Gordon, S., & Nelson, S. (2006). Moving beyond the virtue script in nursing: Creating a knowledge-based identity for nurses. In S. Nelson & S. Gordon (Eds.), *The complexities of care: Nursing reconsidered* (pp. 13–29). Ithaca, NY: Cornell University Press.

Gottlieb, L.N., & Gottlieb, B. (2007). The developmental/health framework within the McGill model of nursing: "Laws of nature" guiding whole person care. *Advances in Nursing Science, 30*(1), E43–E57.

Hartrick Doane, G., & Varcoe, C. (2015). *How to nurse: Relational inquiry with individuals and families in changing health and health care contexts*. Baltimore, MD: Lippincott Williams & Wilkins.

Jones, T., Wear, D., & Friedman, L.D. (Eds.). (2014). *Health humanities reader*. New Brunswick, NJ: Rutgers University Press.

Kleinman, A. (1988). *The illness narratives: Suffering, healing and the human condition*. New York, NY: Basic Books.

Kumagi, A.K. (2008). A conceptual framework for the use of illness narratives in medical education. *Academic Medicine, 83*(7), 653–658.

Massing, M. (2019). Are the humanities history? *New York Review of Books*, 2 April 2019. Retrieved from www.nybooks.com/daily/2019/04/02/are-the-humanities-history/

Neumann, M., Edelhäuser, F., Tauschel, D., Fischer, M.R., Wirtz, M., Woopen, C., Haramati, A., & Scheffer, C. (2011). Empathy decline and its reasons: A systematic review of studies with medical students and residents. *Academic Medicine, 86*(8), 996–1009. doi: 10.1097/ACM.0b013e318221e615

Nussbaum, M.C. (2010). *Not for profit: Why democracy needs the humanities*. Princeton, NJ: Princeton University Press.

Pellegrino, E.D. (1974). Educating the humanist physician: An ancient ideal reconsidered. *Journal of the American Medical Association, 227*(11), 1288–1294.

Risjord, M. (2010). *Nursing knowledge: Science, practice, and philosophy*. Chichester, UK: Wiley-Blackwell.

Robb, A.J.P., & Murray, R. (1992). Medical humanities in nursing: Thought provoking? *Journal of Advanced Nursing, 17*, 1182–1187.

Small, H. (2013). *The value of the humanities*. Oxford, UK: Oxford University Press.

Sullivan, E.J. (1996). Are the humanities still relevant in nursing today? *Journal of Professional Nursing, 12*(5), 267.

Taylor, C. (2007). *A secular age*. Cambridge, MA: Belknap Harvard.

Warner, J.H. (2011). The humanizing power of medical history: Responses to biomedicine in the 20th century United States. *Medical Humanities, 37*, 91–96. doi: 10.1136/medhum-2011-010034

2 Nursing and humanities

History and uses

There is no organized body of work that can neatly be brought together under the heading of nursing humanities. It is not like medical humanities, where it is possible simply to go to that stream in the discipline of medicine and to investigate what is there (a wide stream to be sure, but it has defined edges). There is however a rich history of nurses making use of the humanities, in education, research, and philosophy to make sense of what it is we do, and to communicate it in its dynamic and multivalent fullness. In this chapter, I outline the major ways in which humanities have been taken up by nurses. The first section is about the major ways in which humanities have been used in education. The following sections consider history and philosophy as humanities disciplines that have been taken up to understand and explicate nursing itself. The final section is about the rich discussion in nursing literature of related terms, art, aesthetics, and craft to try to capture nursing in its living movement.

Humanities in nurse education

Education is the obvious place to start. There is an extensive nursing literature about using the humanities in nursing education, including many reports of using different kinds of material from the humanities in teaching, whether in a single project or throughout a programme. There has also been extensive theoretical discussion of the uses and goals of humanities in nurse education. Nurse educators have turned to fiction, memoir, poetry, drama, dance, film, photography, paintings, sculpture – the whole gamut of expressive art forms – in search of ways of enhancing learning for student nurses. The impetus behind turning to artistic modes of expression is not to prettify dry lectures, or to add some diversionary entertainment (though they might do those things too), but to prompt and provoke students, cognitively and affectively, towards what it means to engage with other people, to bring into awareness the values, outlooks, feelings, ideas of others while under the aegis of providing good nursing care.

A good introduction to the topic is still a volume by Valiga and Bruderle (1997), two American nurse educators. In their introduction, they stress the integrative potential of the humanities to show, and to stimulate reflection, on the multivalent experience of affective recognition and response, and critical thinking that occur during events of nursing care. One of their themes, which recurs across disciplines within the health humanities, is the presence of ambiguity and unpredictability, in which decisions have to be made using incomplete information of various kinds in the moment. In providing a guide for nurse educators in bringing humanities into their teaching, they take an inclusive stance towards disciplinary expertise in the humanities, as long as the use of material is guided by the goal of educating nursing students for effective practice.

The bulk of the book consists of chapters about categories of humanities resources, and about topics in which the humanities might be a good fit. The category chapters include literature, film and television, and the fine arts, in which they include visual art as well as performance arts. The topic chapters each start with a concise account of working theories in each area, followed by suggestions of relevant resources. Topic areas include ageing, assessment, death and loss, diversity, family dynamics, and health and illness. One of the themes that runs through these chapters is plurality, in theoretical perspectives, in forms of knowledge for practice, and in the sheer variety of human experience within fundamental aspects of being human like caring or family life. In a couple of respects, the book has dated over 25 years. Suggestions of specific works for use in the classroom often reflect trends from the 1990s, particularly in mass media such as TV programmes or pop music. Since it appeared a few years before the internet age, we are now in a transformed world of access to sources, not to mention means of bringing them into the classroom. If one wanted to use Edvard Munch's painting "The Sick Child" for example, it only takes a moment to find the image online.

Another edited volume on the theme of art and aesthetics in nursing, by Chinn and Watson (1994), has some common ground with Valiga and Bruderle. But whereas the latter is wholly directed towards teaching practice, in Chinn and Watson chapters about application are mixed with theoretical discussions, which are taken up in the section on art and aesthetics later in this chapter. However, the volume does contain practical chapters by different authors about aspects of art in nursing, including writing practice narratives as a form of reflection (Maeve, 1994; Vezeau, 1994), using painting in paediatric nursing (Breunig, 1994), and introducing an artist-in-residence programme in a hospital (Rockwood Lane & Graham-Pole, 1994).

Across the range of nursing literature, there are many descriptions of freestanding initiatives by instructors employing a range of humanities resources, teaching about a range of topics or populations. Approaches include having students watch films (Cappiello & Vroman, 2011), or study paintings in an art gallery (Frei, Alvarez, & Alexander, 2010), then reflect on how they were affected by the experiences depicted. Another example is a study I led with a multidisciplinary team, from nursing, medicine, and English, to explore students' experiences with reading a novel as part of a clinical practicum course (McCaffrey et al., 2017). The students were working with older adults in assisted living or nursing home facilities. Two of their clinical instructors assigned them to read a novel called *Exit Lines* (Barfoot, 2009) that recounted the inner lives and relationships of a group of people who had moved into a new assisted living facility in Ontario, Canada. In small groups at the end of the semester, students joined in facilitated discussion about connections between the novel and what they had experienced in practice. Later, we recruited students to take part in a focus group to share their ideas about the whole experience.

In other reports, instructors had students participate in their own creation of a work, for example writing poetry individually (Coleman & Willis, 2015), or a drama as a group (Deeny et al., 2001). The target topics for these projects include mental health (McKie & Naysmith, 2014), death and dying (Deeny et al., 2001), or qualities of care such as empathy (Özcan, Bilgin, & Eracar, 2011). Many of the published papers are accounts of projects, without any layer of research design or evaluation. Outcomes are thus often given only in terms of student feedback, a common theme of which is that some students liked this kind of approach more than others. In one way, that only expresses a truism about learning styles, and students having mixed reactions to most things they find in the classroom. Beyond that, it invites further questions about what it is that some students respond to positively, and others resist. What is there in how humanities are used that might expand their acceptance and positive reception among students?

There are some examples of research studies of humanities in the classroom, mostly qualitative but occasionally quantitative (Wikström, 2003). With the usual provisos about qualitative research that the sample sizes are mostly small, and the context localized, they show a wide spread of different kinds of humanities resources being used in teaching a variety of topics in nursing.

Although varied in some ways, there are a number of commonalities throughout the descriptions of humanities in nurse education. Some of these are basics of pedagogy, for example that there need to be clearly defined learning outcomes, which might be a blend of cognitive, affective, or sensory learning. One of the hallmarks of humanities, however, which makes it of such value, is that it is rarely uncomplicatedly cognitive as in the learning of facts, or even of critical reasoning within limits of putting together discrete pieces of data. Humanities often involve higher-level cognitive skills of evaluation and creation, in terms of Bloom's taxonomy (University of Waterloo, n.d.). They readily demand affective learning skills of valuing and organization that are directly applicable to human interactions in practice.

Because humanities are used to examine complex, multivalent, and value-laden aspects of human experience they grant access to reflective, open ended, discursive styles of learning. Following from this, a frequent structure of application of humanities in the classroom is the application of, for example, a piece of literature or artwork, to a given topic, so that students have to study the material, then produce ideas about the topic, in light of the material, through some form of guided reflection. Reflection might be required as an individual written assignment or often as group discussion since students have a shared experience of the same material, even though their personal responses will vary.

Another principle that emerges from looking at different examples of educational application of humanities is that they can draw on different levels of participation from students: reading a novel, or writing a short story; hearing and reading a poem, or writing a haiku; watching a film, or making a video; looking at a famous painting, or drawing a cartoon. Humanities offer many different ways for students to be productive and to deepen reflective thinking through trying out modes of expression that might feel uncomfortable but which reach into new ways of looking at a topic.

Using the humanities, as with any pedagogic medium, requires planning, commitment, and knowledge on the part of the educator. The primary goal of humanities in nurse education is that students learn something about nursing, so that planning any specific exercise needs to work back from that goal:

> One does not need to be an expert in literature, sculpture, music, poetry, or drama to use them as tools to facilitate the learning of nursing concepts. What one *does* need, however, is an openness of mind, an appreciation of the art of nursing as well as the science, and a willingness to take risks and use new approaches to stimulate learning and a love of nursing.
>
> (Valiga & Bruderle, 1997, pp. 16–17)

At the same time, it is important to remember that there is more to the humanities than a love of poetry or the arts. They are also academic disciplines with their own set of skills and knowledge. Hearing a good English instructor analyse a text is like watching an expert chef deftly fillet a fish. Part of the team in our novel study (McCaffrey et al., 2017) was just such an instructor, who led one of the small group discussions about the novel at the end of the practice placement. In written feedback, several of those in her group commented that they were surprised to find just how much insight they gained from her expert questioning and suggestions: insight into the novel and through the novel into the lives of older adults in assisted living, and ultimately into their own attitudes and behaviour. There are abundant opportunities for educators in nursing to use the humanities in their teaching, and additionally opportunities for creative and rich interdisciplinary collaborations.

There are also recurrent questions or problems that arise. One is that many authors note that not all students like this kind of exercise. When we conducted the focus group with students in our novel study, one of their first comments was to point out that they had volunteered for the study because they liked the exercise – many of their friends, they told us, had found it unnecessary and had not engaged with it (McCaffrey et al., 2017). One answer is to say, as educators, that we know many students do not like studying statistics, but we still have them do it because we know it is good for you (we are nurses, after all). Another partial answer is to think carefully about whether or not assignments are mandatory or voluntary, and what incentives we give for completing them. In the case of our novel reading, it was part of a pass/fail course in which the primary concern was competence in practice, so it was not likely that the instructors were going to fail students for not wanting to read a novel. Also, two instructors took the initiative to introduce the novel, which was an excellent choice for the context, and they conducted the assignment with great skill and enthusiasm – but other groups in the same course did not have to read it, so some of the dislike was based on a sense of unfairly having to do extra reading.

A further question is that of scale and purpose within a broader horizon of a programme or curriculum. Most of the examples given above were small-scale initiatives, within a single class. That speaks to the adaptability of using humanities. A short clip from a sitcom, or a poem of a few lines, can be used to leaven the dough of teaching a subject like pathophysiology. There may not be many instructors who never use the humanities at all in some form, but then there are examples of more systematic integration of humanities into nursing programmes. McKie et al. (2008) describe a module using expressive arts as an option within a nursing degree programme in Scotland. Darbyshire (1994) gives an account of developing, delivering, and evaluating a course on caring through the use of arts and humanities. This approach shows a more serious commitment to the assertion that humanities have a place in the panoply of nursing knowledge. Connected programming would habituate students to bringing a greater diversity of ways of thinking into their formation as nurses.

A vexed question for the humanities in health care, which has garnered a lot of attention in medical humanities, where they have been more deliberately inserted into curricula, is that of evaluation. That is, not evaluation of students for grades, but of whether using humanities has the desired effect on students' knowledge or behaviour. There tend to be two distinct points of view. One, from a purer vision of the value to individuals and society of exposure to art, says that it is more or less impossible to measure the effects of the humanities and is unnecessary anyway. Cultural creativity and appreciation are so deeply embedded in human social life that their value, indeed necessity, speaks for itself even if it cannot be broken down into a one-for-one cause and effect like a pharmaceutical agent. (It is not difficult to parody the desire to measure such things – *The Merchant of Venice* yields a 7 per cent greater increase in empathy than *King Lear* [$p = 0.45$].) On the other side, if humanities content is treated like another kind of intervention, then it should also be measured like one. Ousager and Johannessen (2010) carried out a review of 245 articles about humanities in undergraduate medical education. Although they reported overwhelmingly positive support on the part of authors, they judged that only nine articles showed evidence of long-term effects. Belling (2010) in an editorial response argued that the problem was not in the findings themselves, according to the methodological logic of the review, but one of a category error in basic assumptions. The value of the humanities, she argued, lies precisely in their counterweight to reductionism, in their capacity to countenance uncertainty, and in their "focus ... on the specific and particular, exactly those aspects of human texts that resist reduction" (p. 940). There is a tension between different epistemological assumptions that can be made plain but probably not fully resolved. It is for those working with humanities in health professions' education to make decisions about how they define goals and how they are going to determine degrees of success in achieving them. Those may include statistical measures, survey feedback, or narrative and discursive accounts by students, even artistic productions.

History of nursing

History as a humanities discipline takes nursing as one area of study. Historians might come to nursing from the outside, or nurse scholars trained in methods of historical research might bring an insider perspective (Lewenson & Herrmann, 2008). Amongst other things, studying history is not a bad training in thinking for nurses. As the distinguished historian Margaret MacMillan says, "Historians ... are trained to ask questions, make connections, and collect and examine the evidence" (2009, p. 45), drawing on established knowledge but also able to forge new connections, discover new insights, and challenge old assumptions. History is often disregarded as either irrelevant or merely picturesque, and of little importance in a culture fixed upon the future, progress, and the latest cell phone. Nelson and Gordon (2004) point out the danger in this mindset for nursing, of never properly recognizing the dense, practical skills of nurses in the past, and as a consequence having a thinned out conceptualization of nursing that leaves the profession prey to passing political trends. In another paper, warning against historical amnesia, Nelson (2009) argues that historical study bears witness and is crucial "in the on-going development of identity" (p. 5).

History helps us to take possession of identity formation of groups to which we belong, to debate whatever that might mean, to make informed arguments about preferences for the future. It helps us too, to understand something of other groups, how they see themselves, and why, and how they might respond to us (MacMillan, 2009). History is not merely a repository of past events, though it relies on well-researched evidence, but a continuing reflective process by which we understand ourselves better in light of the past, and in light of the preoccupations we bring to the past. In the twenty-first century, for example, historical study in nursing has turned more towards the daily reality of practice using material resources, than the lives of great nurses (*European Journal for History and Ethics*, 2019; Nelson, 2009; Sandelowski, 2000). The idea that we are historical beings, whether we like it or not, is captured in the hermeneutic philosopher Gadamer's concept of "historically effected consciousness" (1960/2004, p. 336). We are both products of traditions, and actors within them. Our thinking is shaped by the values and beliefs that already exist, say when we enter into a profession like nursing, but those values and beliefs are not static, they go on transforming through networks of interaction with both internal and external forces. To study history is to lift up one's head, to be able to get a clearer view of what is going on around us. For a profession like nursing, whose practitioners have often complained of being invisible or subordinate, history is a valuable resource.

Philosophy of nursing

Nursing is a practical occupation and most nurses, most of the time, are rightly focused on what they need to do in the moment for their patients or clients. But even such a sparse statement invites questions about the proper limits of nursing: occupation versus profession, why patients *or* clients, or something else, not to mention *rightly*? Whether you take the long view, that nursing as we know it today is the latest form of a fundamental aspect of human life, or say that nursing as a defined profession is only about 150 years old, it is important enough and complex enough to provoke serious philosophical consideration. Philosophy, one of the traditional humanities disciplines, has become one forum for humanities permeating nursing even though it is not often explicitly thought of in that way.

Theory, at least in the sense of striving for grand, all-encompassing theories of nursing as such, has in the twenty-first century given ground to philosophy as the vehicle for thinking about nursing. Philosophy is better suited to the task, since it only sets out basic principles, that there are serious questions to be addressed, and that they should be addressed carefully and rigorously, without grand theory's promise of ultimate explanation. Philosophy shows up in graduate level classes providing nursing students with traditions, frameworks, ideas, and lexicons which they can use to deepen and then articulate their understanding of problems they have encountered in the everyday world of health care delivery. Nursing research, embracing both quantitative and qualitative methods, is shot through with philosophical arguments about epistemology, pluralism, value, and rigour, in the cause of methodological strength. Philosophy plays host to competing ideas about the ultimate goals of nursing, about the nature of human beings, or about what we mean by health, science, and caring.

Nurse academics have found certain streams of philosophy to be amenable to the practices and ends of nurses. Science, too often dismissed as anti-holistic, has perhaps not received enough attention philosophically as a diverse and dynamic tradition. In the US, the introduction of the Doctorate of Nursing Practice has brought with it an unequivocal embrace of evidence-based practice, prioritizing statistically verifiable knowledge according to the hierarchy of evidence. Nevertheless, as Dahnke and Dreher (2016) point out in their philosophy of science textbook aimed at DNP students, it is still important that doctoral students understand the philosophical foundations for the knowledge they are expected to use, synthesize, and apply.

The twentieth century philosophical movement of phenomenology has become popular because it appears to provide a systematic route into subjective experience. Phenomenology's offshoot, hermeneutics develops the idea that experience necessarily entails interpreting the world, which offers a further dimension to exploring the significance of communication between people in nursing work. Critical social theory has leverage for many nurses in opening up questions of resource allocation, access, and political structure as they affect nurses and patients in health care systems. Often in association with critical theory, some nurses add post-structuralist ideas about language and discourse to the mix to make x-rays of the skeleton of power relationships in and around nursing (Rodgers, 2005).

As the discipline of nursing has matured and settled into its educational home in universities, so has the self-protective impulse towards establishing an autonomous realm of nursing knowledge and research lessened. Thinkers in nursing are now much more focused on the scope of nursing practice as the source for nursing research, feeding back directly or indirectly into improving practice. Philosophy has accommodated and guided the shift. Mark Risjord (2010), a philosopher who has worked closely with nurses, argues persuasively against a restrictive focus on separate paradigms of qualitative and quantitative research, in favour of thinking of knowledge as a web that is flexible, includes disparate kinds of statements, and is given sense and coherence by application to a question arising in nursing practice.

Nurse theorists have continued to develop accounts of nursing that seek to find ways of describing practice that does justice to the subjective, objective, social, ethical, technical, sensory, cognitive, and emotional (not a definitive list) dimensions of nursing. Benner (1984), one of the pioneers of phenomenology in nursing, elaborated the trajectory of novice to expert, capturing the experience nurses have of becoming so adept at practice that they cease to register much of their decision-making processes. In her more recent work (2011) she has developed the concept of formation to articulate the development of a competent, well-functioning nurse over time, and to use it to make recommendations for pedagogy that brings students purposefully into practice.

Kim (2015) has a complex model of nursing practice, which makes use of philosophy as a constituent of the whole. She delineates "three philosophical orientations [of] ... care ... therapy ... and professional work" (p. 19) as one structure within a comprehensive model. Caring is subordinated to one of these sub-structures, an important part of nursing, but for Kim not a singular essence since nursing also has to include the "instrumental" and "social" (p. 71) orientations of therapy and professional work respectively. Kim's work is representative of a trend towards pluralist and integrative accounts of nursing that are practice-led, but which also require philosophical thinking and language for their expression.

Humanities and nursing research

Philosophy in nursing is strongly connected with research, through graduate level courses in the foundational concepts and assumptions of research methods, and through research methodologies that claim philosophical justification. All research needs to be demonstrably worth doing, but most of the time, in the case of statistical research, its epistemological basis is not considered as worth restating. The value of a particular study is given at the level of the appropriateness of the question, based upon existing literature, on the verifiably correct conduct of the stated method, and the strength of the results. Researchers, however, at least initially ought to understand the foundations upon which their studies are built, hence Dahnke and Dreher's (2016) volume of philosophy of science for nurses.

When it comes to other, qualitative methods, however, researchers claim a much more explicit relationship between philosophical tenets and research methods. Phenomenology as a research method has flourished in nursing because of its attention to "lived experience" and the "lifeworld" of health care environments. Researchers draw a direct line to the work of Husserl in the early twentieth century and his project of describing things fully and precisely through the medium of subjective experience. As a way of getting to a phenomenon like pain, for example, phenomenology has an obvious appeal for nurse researchers who want to produce worthwhile information about what it is like to be on the receiving end of health care (or to be delivering health care). Thinkers who came after Husserl, most notably Heidegger and Merleau-Ponty, are also often cited in nursing studies. Heidegger (1927/1962) challenged Husserl's claim to objectivity by arguing that human beings are so immersed in the world of things and actions, that they are always oriented towards the world in ways of which they are not consciously aware. This too, has appeal to researchers in a practice profession, where institutional and professional values, as well as personal disposition, are at play in the most routine of situations. Merleau-Ponty (1945/2012) thematized embodiment, writing a massive phenomenology of what it is to be a human being living in, and experiencing the world through, a sensing body. Again, his work has obvious interest for nurses coming from a practice of caring for bodies, even in the case of mental health, bodies that express feelings through movement, that have to occupy space in controlled environments, and bodies that digest psychotropic drugs. Phenomenological research has come in for a lot of criticism, not least from philosopher John Paley (2016) who has written extensively on nursing matters. One of his arguments is that the connection between philosophy and research process is not nearly as close or as logical as phenomenological researchers have claimed, leading to results that may have some descriptive interest but cannot claim to get to the supposed essence of a phenomenon.

Hermeneutic philosophy emerged out of phenomenology, first through Heidegger, then Gadamer in Germany and Ricoeur in France. Hermeneutics, which means interpretation, is a philosophy of how it is that human beings come to understand their experience and make sense of the world as a joined-up process. Hermeneutic thinkers place a lot of emphasis on language as the medium of understanding, and on history and culture as the conditions of shared experience by which individuals also enter social life. With its attention to language, hermeneutics in research is invariably used to explore questions that centre on interactions between nurses and others, and with its insistence on context, it can avoid the narrow focus on reported experience alone that can limit phenomenology (Moules, McCaffrey, Field, & Lang, 2015).

Narrative inquiry is another qualitative research method, based on the assumption that as human beings we understand ourselves as continuing entities through connected narratives about who we are, and our place in the world

(Clandinin, 2013). Narrative self-understanding pulls us into the world and is made up of threads of "the social, cultural, familial, linguistic, and institutional narratives within which individuals' experiences were, and are, constituted, shaped, expressed, and enacted" (Clandinin, 2013, p. 18). Narrative inquiry shares a belief in the importance of narrative with narrative medicine, mentioned in the previous chapter, and has some common ground with the historical identity formation as studied by historians. It is distinct, however, in taking up narrative as the basis for research, by allowing individuals or groups, in collaboration with researchers, to articulate the sources and consequences of their storied selves.

In arts-based research, art forms might not just be the subject matter of research, but themselves become part of the research process (Barone & Eisler, 2012; Knowles & Cole, 2008). Arts-based methodologies draw upon the traditional place of art as expressive of cultural meanings and values to use art forms in a more directed way to examine chosen areas of experience. Research can make use of performing arts, visual arts, plastic arts, or literary arts to create new knowledge.

Nursing, art, and aesthetics

First, some dictionary definitions:

> **Aesthetics**: (Noun) The philosophy of the beautiful or of art; a system of principles for the appreciation of the beautiful.
>
> **Aesthetic**: (Adjective) Of or pertaining to the appreciation or criticism of the beautiful or of art.
>
> **Art**: 1. Skill as the result of knowledge or practice. Technical or professional skill. 2. The learning of the schools; scholarship [historical] 3. The application of skill according to aesthetic principles, esp. in the production of visible works of imagination, imitation, or design (painting, sculpture, architecture, etc.); skilful execution of workmanship as an object in itself.
>
> **Craft**: 2. Skill, art: ability in planning or constructing; ingenuity, dexterity. 5. An art, trade, or profession requiring special skill or knowledge, esp. manual dexterity.
>
> (*Shorter Oxford Dictionary*, 1993)

One strand in nursing philosophy that demands attention, since I am talking about arts and humanities in relation to nursing, is the discussion of aesthetics, including a related debate about the art or craft (or neither) of nursing. Aesthetics as a theme was raised by Carper (1978) in her influential paper, where she names it as one of the four ways of knowing in nursing. What Carper says, what she does not say, and what she might have said has been a source of discussion of aesthetics in nursing ever since. Talk of the *art of nursing*, however, goes back to Florence Nightingale in this quotation that appears frequently in the nursing aesthetics literature:

> Nursing is an art and, if it is to be made an art, requires as exclusive a devotion, as hard a preparation, as any painter's or sculptor's work, for what is the having to do with dead canvas or cold marble compared with having to do with the living body, the temple of God's spirit? It is one of the fine arts; I had almost said, the finest of the fine arts.
>
> (McDonald, 1868/2004, pp. 291–292)

The historical definition of art (# 2) at the head of this section may partly explain Nightingale's employment of the term. Medicine, as one of the schools of the medieval university, was traditionally counted among the arts before the Enlightenment separation of arts and sciences, hence "the art of medicine" has a long ancestry prior to more modern attributions. Perhaps Nightingale had in mind the art of nursing as a counterpoint to the art of medicine lending it an air of historic rootedness. It is worth noting too, that the famous Nightingale quotation comes in a piece of writing that is part elegy for a "pioneer of workhouse nursing" (McDonald, 1868/2004, p. 290) who had died young, and part rallying cry to Nightingale's vision of religiously motivated, yet non-sectarian nurses drawn from all social classes. Immediately before the comments about art, she praised the deceased nurse's work ethic and organizational skills, for "How can any undervalue business habits?, as if anything could be done without them" (p. 291). It is worth keeping in mind, that Nightingale in this passage was not delivering a definition of nursing, but treating it as a multifaceted practice.

Carper's motivation for writing her paper, as she explained in a later interview (Eisenhauer, 2015), was to counter what she saw as an over-emphasis on science as all that was necessary in nurse education. She mentions in the same interview that at one stage in her career she set up a nursing programme in a liberal arts college, where she collaborated with colleagues in the liberal arts and humanities. She also disclaims the suggestion her work should be considered as a theory, instead describing it as "a cultural or intellectual philosophy of nursing" (p. 78). These later reflections are helpful in framing the way she brought aesthetics into her discussion of nursing. She was comfortable with the idea that the arts and humanities had some bearing on nursing, and was trying to capture aspects of nursing that were not – and still are not – as easily articulated as the rational application of evidence.

In her original paper, Carper proposed that aesthetic experience includes attention to what is "specific and unique" (1978, p. 18), and "transformation of … the patient's behavior – into a direct, nonmediated perception of what is significant in it …" (p. 17). She included empathy as "an important mode in the aesthetic pattern of knowing" (p. 19) as a way of increasing the nurse's available range of helpful responses to an individual patient. Thus, she was using aesthetic knowing to get at elements of nursing care that involve subjectivity, affect, and imagination.

Since art and aesthetics entered the nursing lexicon, they have continued to be debated in the literature. Chinn (1994) touched on therapeutic uses of art but also on "nursing as an art form" (p. viii) and "aesthetic inquiry" (p. viii) as a broad category outside of the reach of standard scientific knowledge. Johnson (1994), in the same issue of *Advances in Nursing Science*, reviewed 41 articles about art in nursing and derived five recurrent themes from them. The first two themes pertain to meaning, in the nurse's ability to make sense of patient encounters and to establish a connection with the patient. The third is about skills, the fourth about rational planning, and the fifth moral conduct. These are genuine and important aspects of nursing practice that relate more to art in the sense of skilful practice than artistic expression. Johnson's breakdown is a useful discussion of attempts to get at what nursing practice is like, and what it demands of the practitioner in addition to scientific knowledge and technical competence.

Chinn and Watson (1997) edited a book devoted to *Arts and Aesthetics in Nursing*, published by the National League for Nursing in the United States. Their introductory chapter is a manifesto for the art of nursing, for art as a form of spiritual expression, and for caring as both, culminating in a call that:

> Nursing must be radically reimagined if it is to restore its caring-healing fine art and the view of mind/body/spirit unity that is the basis of its practice. In this revision, nursing art and spirituality – the sacred – need to be seen again as one.
>
> (1997, p. xvi)

I find the conflation of art, spirituality, caring, and nursing too loose to be helpful. None of these terms necessitates any of the others, except in the conventional association between caring and nursing, and even then a lot of work is needed to pin down "caring" with any degree of precision. Of course, all of the terms can be linked somehow, since they are all so open to numerous interpretations. There are some more prosaic observations in Chinn and Watson's account, for example, like Carper, finding aesthetic qualities in the physical activity of nursing, which "… includes direction, force, balance, and rhythm" (p. xvi). Idealizing art, however, covers over art as provocation, as social criticism, as showing the uglier aspects of human life, or as expressing inner conflict disappears behind veils of spiritual knowing.

Wainwright (1999; 2000) drew attention to the difference senses of the word art and the confusion that can arise from a term that holds such varied meanings. He is happy with the more general sense of art as skilled human activity, but also notes that this sense does then not add much to talking about nursing practice. de Raeve (1998) also has reservations about the art of nursing, which she extends to a discussion of Carper's aesthetics. She does recognize the need that prompted the line of argument in the first place:

> One can have considerable sympathy with this view that there is an important, underdiscussed and under-rated dimension to nursing that cannot

be captured by scientific language or understanding, but two questions remain: is it knowledge; and is it to do with aesthetics?

(p. 402)

An alternative to nursing as an art, which makes a less sustained appearance in the literature, is nursing as a craft. Two of the dictionary definitions of craft above already include art, and "art, trade, or profession requiring special skill or knowledge" is broad enough to include nursing. For Edwards (1998), however, the arts/craft distinction centres on the ends of an activity, which for craft are circumscribed and known in advance, for example mending a shoe. If art is intended to capture the role of imagination and adaptability to changing circumstances, then to call nursing a craft would fall short. Phil Barker, a strong advocate of the therapeutic scope of mental health nursing, puts craft at the centre of his ideas about nursing. He sees craft as the potent blending of "both knowledge (science) and aesthetics (art)" (2009, p. 7) in order to meet the needs of another person. The known goal or product of craft is what makes the term more, not less, appropriate to the purposeful, other-oriented practice of nursing where the goal is caring. In context, Barker's use of the term craft is part of his powerful advocacy for a conduct of mental health nursing that demands therapeutic engagement with service users, supporting them in working towards their own forms of working with "problems in living" (p. 3). Barker is keen to stress the practical realities of mental health nursing, of what nurses do or do not do to care for others, and craft conveys this better than art as a metaphor. Like art, however, it is a metaphor that takes some work to find the fit with nursing since craft has connotations of manipulating objects using relatively simple tools, whereas in nursing the outcome of caring is not an object that can be simply handed over from craftsperson to customer, and at times, if not so often in mental health nursing, it involves sophisticated technology. While craft serves to emphasize the human-scale interactions that are so vital to nursing, it also tends to obscure the technical and scientific elements that are also necessary.

More recently, authors have highlighted an integrative function that they find in Carper's aesthetic pattern of knowing (Archibald, 2012; Hartrick-Doane & Varcoe, 2015). Again, this is a perspective that reflects a common, and important theme in modern writing about nursing, of how to talk about all the multifarious things that are going on in nursing activity *at the same time.* One of the reasons that Carper's paper has resonated with nurses for so long, in spite of all the critique it has received, is surely that she effectively named this problem of talking about something nurses know from their own working lives. How to talk about integration as experienced, or witnessed, in practice is difficult, and aesthetics is one way of trying to capture it, even though it falls short against conventional usage of the term.

The discussion of art and aesthetics in nursing reveals a desire to find good ways of expressing what nursing practice is like, to capture its distinct blend of activity, interpersonal relationship, engagement with health and illness, with objective knowledge, and affective, subjective experience. If aesthetics or art, for some commentators, and for me, does not seem a very good fit for all of this, it is not because there is not a phenomenon that demands attention and analysis. "The art and science of nursing" is a phrase that comes easily to nurses and reflects an assumption or perhaps a deeply felt need that scientific thinking and technical skills do not encompass the full world of nursing. Quite what we mean when we say art in the context of nursing is not easy to define, and maybe that is the point. It is a philosophical question, open to interpretation and dispute, but a question that has life because it touches on the evanescent, unrepeatable interchanges between peoples' lives that take place within a situation – that of nursing care – which is in other ways highly defined and delimited.

Conclusion

Looking at the uses of humanities in nursing education, philosophy, and research has shown the substance of the relationship between nursing and humanities. Humanities constitute a vital part of nursing knowledge, and can address aspects of nursing practice that are not easy to encapsulate in a single category. Longstanding and continuing debates about art, aesthetics and craft in nursing are motivated by a need to capture experience that is at once evanescent and deeply felt. Humanities, thought of as a set of perspectives and disciplinary skills, hold resources to carry on the endeavour of showing the what, why, and how of nursing care as fulsomely as possible.

References

Archibald, M.M. (2012). The holism of aesthetic knowing in nursing. *Nursing Philosophy*, *13*, 179–188.

Austgard, K. (2006). The aesthetic experience of nursing. *Nursing Philosophy*, *7*, 11–19.

Barker, P. (2009). The nature of nursing. In P. Barker (Ed.), *Psychiatric and mental health nursing: The craft of caring* (2nd ed.; pp. 3–11). London, UK: Hodder Arnold.

Barfoot, J. (2009). *Exit lines*. Toronto, ON, Canada: Vintage Canada.

Barone, T., & E.W. Eisner. (2012). *Arts based research.* Thousand Oaks, CA: Sage.

Belling, C. (2010). Sharper instruments: On defending the humanities in undergraduate medical education. *Academic Medicine*, *85*, 938–940.

Benner, P. (1984). *From novice to expert*. Menlo Park, CA: Addison-Wesley.

Benner, P. (2011). Formation in professional education: An examination of the relationship between theories of meaning and theories of the self. *Journal of Medicine and Philosophy*, *36*, 342–353. doi: 10.1093/jmp/jhr030

Breunig, K. (1994). The art of painting meets the art of nursing. In P.L. Chinn & J. Watson (Eds.), *Art and aesthetics in nursing* (pp. 67–90). New York, NY: National League for Nursing Press.

Cappiello, J.D., & Vroman, K. (2011). Bring the popcorn: Using film to teach sexual and reproductive health. *International Journal of Nursing Education Scholarship*, *8*(1), 1–17. doi: 10.2202/1548-923X.2133

Carper, B.A. (1978). Fundamental patterns of knowing in nursing. *Advances in Nursing Science*, *1*(1), 13–24.

Chinn, P.L. (1994). Art and aesthetics in nursing. *Advances in Nursing Science, 17*(1), viii.

Chinn, P.L., & Watson, J. (Eds.). (1994). *Art and aesthetics in nursing.* New York, NY: National League for Nursing Press.

Clandinin, D.J. (2013). *Engaging in narrative inquiry.* Walnut Creek, CA: Left Coast Press.

Coleman, D., & Willis, D.S. (2015). Reflective writing: The student nurse's perspective on reflective writing and poetry writing. *Nurse Education Today, 35*(7), 906–911. doi. org/10.1016/j.nedt.2015.02.018

Dahnke, M.D., & Dreher, H.M. (2016). *Philosophy of science for nursing practice: Concepts and applications* (2nd ed.). New York, NY: Springer.

Darbyshire, P. (1994). Understanding caring through arts and humanities: A medical/ nursing humanities approach to promoting alternative experiences of thinking and learning. *Journal of Advanced Nursing, 19*, 856–863.

de Raeve, L. (1998). The art of nursing: An aesthetics? *Nursing Ethics, 5*(5), 402–411.

Deeny, P., Johnson, A., Boore, J., Leyden, C., & McCaughan, E. (2001). Drama as an experiential technique in learning how to cope with dying patients and their families. *Teaching in Higher Education, 6*(1), 99–112. doi: 10.1080/13562510124223

Edwards, S.D. (1998). The art of nursing. *Nursing Ethics, 5*(5), 393–400.

Eisenhauer, E.R. (2015). An interview with Dr. Barbara A. Carper. *Advances in Nursing Science, 38*(2), 73–82.

European Journal for Nursing History and Ethics. (2019). Retrieved from www.enhe.eu

Frei, J., Alvarez, S.E., & Alexander, M.B. (2010). Ways of seeing: Using the visual arts in nursing education. *Journal of Nursing Education, 49*(12), 672–676.

Gadamer, H.G. (1960/2004). *Truth and method* (J. Weinsheimer & D.G. Marshall, Trans.). New York, NY: Continuum.

Hartrick-Doane, G., & Varcoe, C. (2015). *How to nurse: Relational inquiry with individuals and families in challenging health and health care contexts.* Philadelphia, PA: Wolters Kluwer.

Heidegger, M. (1927/1962). *Being and time.* New York: HarperCollins.

Johnson, J. (1994). A dialectical examination of nursing art. *Advances in Nursing Science, 17*(1), 1–14.

Kim, H.S. (2015). *The essence of nursing practice: Philosophy and perspective.* New York, NY: Springer.

Knowles, J.G., & Cole, A.L. (Eds.). (2008). *Handbook of the arts in qualitative research.* Thousand Oaks, CA: Sage.

Lewenson, S.B., & Herrmann, E.K. (Eds.). (2008). *Capturing nursing history: A guide to historical methods in research.* New York, NY: Springer.

MacMillan, M. (2009). *The uses and abuses of history.* Toronto, ON, Canada: Penguin Canada.

Maeve, M.K. (1994). Coming to moral consciousness through the art of nursing narratives. In P.L. Chinn & J. Watson (Eds.), *Art and aesthetics in nursing* (pp. 67–90). New York, NY: National League for Nursing Press.

McCaffrey, G., Venturato, L., Patterson, J.D., Langille, J., Jackson, R., & Rosenal, T. (2017). Bringing a novel to practice: An interpretive study of reading a novel in an undergraduate nursing practicum course. *Nursing Education in Practice, 24*, 84–89. doi.org/10.1016/j.nepr.2017.04.001

McDonald, L. (Ed.). (2004). *Florence Nightingale on public health care: Collected works of Florence Nightingale, Vol. 6.* Waterloo, ON, Canada: Wilfred Laurier University Press.

McKie, A., Adams, V., Gass, J.P., & Macduff, C. (2008). Windows and mirrors: Reflections of a module team teaching the arts in nurse education. *Nurse Education in Practice, 8*, 156–164.

McKie, A., & Naysmith, S. (2014). Promoting critical perspectives in mental health nursing education. *Journal of Psychiatric and Mental Health Nursing, 21*, 128–137. doi: 10.1111/jpm.12061

Merleau-Ponty, M. (2012). Phenomenology of perception (D.A. Landes, Trans.). New York, NY: Routledge.

Moules, N.J., McCaffrey, G., Field, J., & Laing, C. (2015). *Conducting hermeneutic research: From philosophy to practice.* New York, NY: Peter Lang.

Nelson, S. (2009). Historical amnesia and its consequences – the need to build histories of practice. *Texto Contexto Enferm, Florianópolis, 18*(4), 781–787.

Nelson, S., & Gordon, S. (2004). The rhetoric of rupture: Nursing as a practice with a history? *Nursing Outlook, 52*, 255–261.

Ousager, J., & Johannessen, H. (2010). Humanities in undergraduate medical education: A literature review. *Academic Medicine, 85*, 988–998.

Özcan, N.K., Bilgin, H., & Eracar, N. (2011). The use of expressive methods for developing empathic skills. *Issues in Mental Health Nursing, 32*(2), 131–136. doi: 10.3109/01612840.2010.534575

Paley, J. (2016). *Phenomenology as qualitative research: A critical analysis of meaning attribution.* Abingdon, UK: Routledge.

Risjord, M. (2010). *Nursing knowledge: Science, practice, and philosophy.* Chichester, UK: Wiley-Blackwell.

Rockwood Lane, M.T., & Graham-Pole, J. (1994). The power of creativity in healing: A practice model demonstrating the links between the creative arts and the art of nursing. In P.L. Chinn & J. Watson (Eds.), *Art and aesthetics in nursing* (pp. 67–90). New York, NY: National League for Nursing Press.

Rodgers, B.L. (2005). *Developing nursing knowledge: Philosophical traditions and influences.* Philadelphia, PA: Lippincott Williams & Wilkins.

Shorter Oxford dictionary. Oxford, UK: Clarendon.

Sandelowski, M. (2000). *Devices and desires: Gender, technology, and American nursing.* Chapel Hill, NC: University of North Carolina Press.

University of Waterloo. (n.d.). *Bloom's taxonomy.* Waterloo, ON, Canada: Author. Retrieved from https://uwaterloo.ca/centre-for-teaching-excellence/teaching-resources/teaching-tips/planning-courses-and-assignments/course-design/blooms-taxonomy

Valiga, T.M., & Bruderle, E.R. (1997). *Using the arts and humanities to teach nursing: A creative approach.* New York, NY: Springer.

Vezeau, T.M. (1994). Narrative in nursing practice and education. In P.L. Chinn & J. Watson (Eds.), *Art and aesthetics in nursing* (pp. 67–90). New York, NY: National League for Nursing Press.

Wainwright, P. (1999). The art of nursing. *International Journal of Nursing Studies, 36*, 379–385.

Wainwright, P. (2000). Towards an aesthetics of nursing. *Journal of Advanced Nursing, 32*(3), 750–756.

Wikström, B.M. (2003). A picture of a work of art as an empathy teaching strategy in nurse education complementary to theoretical knowledge. *Journal of Professional Nursing, 19*(1), 49–54.

3 What is nursing?

It seems late to be coming to the question of what is nursing? Surely it is obvious, certainly to the many nurses in the world who go about their daily work without troubling about the question, or to those who come to them with needs that they reasonably expect to be addressed. However, the question remains worth considering because the answer is not static. Nursing now is not the same as it was when I began my career over 30 years ago and certainly not the same as it was in Florence Nightingale's time, let alone pre-Nightingale. One feature of the past 50 years or so is that nurse education has moved into colleges and universities, prompting a great deal of thought among the new class of nurse academics about nursing and their place in it. Much of this thinking has identified, and arguably perpetuated a division between the relational and the technical, the caring and the scientific, the subjective and the objective. There are numerous terms that can be placed on either side of an assumed line that runs through the existential world of nurses. There have been various approaches to the division; theoreticians who have taken up one side or the other with varying degrees of fervour and others who have sought different kinds of pluralism or accommodation. Writers about nursing theory have for the most part moved beyond the attempts of the 1970s and 1980s to come up with a juggernaut grand theory that would encompass all of nursing in favour of more local and varied perspectives that attend to questions arising from nursing practice.

The question I am asking about the nature of nursing is not looking for a theoretical, prescriptive answer, but for some understanding of the underlying characteristics of nursing that make some sense of the enduring division and that accounts for it not as some flaw in modern nursing, but as a characteristic. In this chapter, I look at nursing in two complementary ways: first, from a naturalist perspective thinking of nursing as one kind of human activity that expresses evolved human drives. Second, from an historical perspective, seeing contemporary nursing as a conditioned, cultural phenomenon.

Naturalized nursing

The origins of the word "nurse" suggest something ancient and fundamental in human life (Gottlieb & Gottlieb, 2007). Nurse derives from the Latin *nutrix* meaning "wet nurse", from *nutrire* "to suckle" with the additional connotations of nourish and, later, nurture (Online Etymology Dictionary, 2019). It is rooted in the primal relationship between mother and infant, providing the means of life and growth. Etymology is not destiny however. The origin of the English word does root nursing in fundamental care and it is of course, gendered. However, in its evolution, it is the structure of a caring relationship that has remained important. By contrast, the French word for nurse, *infirmièr/e*, has masculine and feminine forms, but its meaning has to do with the situation of the one being cared for, the infirm patient. In the sixteenth century, the word nurse took on its more general modern meaning of one who cares for the sick, extending the sense of a relationship of providing sustenance for another. The basic structure of care is not unique to nursing, but it is one of the hallmarks of nursing that is carried in the word itself. Modern nursing writers have expended a great deal of energy in trying to work out the implications of the caring relationship and to bring it into alignment with the vastly complex and varied activities that now come under the rubric of nursing. Strategies have ranged from creating a new science of caring (Eriksson, 2002), to advising moving away from the preoccupation with caring because it represents an anti-scientific gesture that undermines the credibility of nursing (Paley, 2002).

The felt association between nursing and caring, however, is not incidental or peripheral however difficult it might be to rein it in as a discrete, quantifiable entity. Nursing care is a compound term in such everyday use as to be almost tautologous, except that in the addition of the word "care" lies the implication of action, of practice, of all the things nurses do to bring nursing into expression, to make concrete the living identity of the nurse in the world. Hence the "care plan", much debated over the course of my career as to specific form, value or purpose, but nonetheless persisting as a formulation of the idea that the nurse needs to be able to articulate what she is going to *do* to enact care. Caring as a category of activities within human societies is about doing for others. It is an expression of the affiliative drives in human beings, the basic prosocial inclinations that allow groups of people to live, survive, cooperate, and flourish together.

Basic drives

Mary Midgley is a British philosopher who has written extensively about the role of sociability and cooperation in human evolution – and in other species, for that matter – in contrast to accounts that prioritize self-interest and competition as the drivers of evolution. For Midgley, "… we are actually earthly organisms, framed to interact continually with the complex ecosystems of which we are a tiny part. For us, *bonds* are not just awkward restraints. They are lifelines" (2010, p. 124). Social bonds and "feelings of fellowship" (p. 31) are intrinsic to human life, such that generosity and altruism are natural impulses. Parent-child attachment is one form of bond, which not only protects the vulnerable infant, but lays the foundation for social development. Developments in cognitive neuroscience have confirmed the significance of early attachment at the organic level of healthy brain development, and have helped to delineate the potential negative effects of poor attachment in individuals' capacity in later life to live well in relationship with others (Center on the Developing Child, 2007). Parental attachment comes back to the archetypal mother-child nurturance buried in the word nurse. Nursing is an expression of deep prosocial drives, rooted perhaps in early attachment but extended out to a broader altruism.

Midgley is not, however, arguing that the vision of individual competition derived from Darwin is simply wrong, nor that by the exercise of moral will, we can overcome selfish impulses and choose to live for others. She is aiming to provide a corrective to versions of evolutionary thought that put individual competition at the centre of human life and to argue instead that we are made up of conflicting drives. Morality arises out of inner conflict, not as an external restraint, but as a way of managing the "chronic friction" (p. 27) inside human life. Acknowledging that humans have different drives and that we have to manage the consequences, in our day-to-day individual lives, and at higher levels of social organization, gives a very broad framework for trying to make sense of human activities, including nursing. If nursing is associated with caring, that comes as no surprise. If individual nurses do not seem very caring on occasions, that ought to be no surprise either, even if seen as a problem to be managed. Nursing as a broad category is underpinned by prosocial drives, but no individual is motivated exclusively, all the time by prosocial drives.

Locating nursing within a broad account of human motivation and behaviour helps to frame the need for nursing as a broad category of caring activity but cannot account for its specific features at a point in historical time, or in a certain kind of society. Nursing, like all complex human activities, is mediated culturally and historically.

Historical and cultural formation

Modern nursing emerged in the mid-nineteenth century in response to new needs for a class of carer who could keep up with developments in medical science, serve the public, and work in institutions. Bringing nurses together into a collective group demanded standardization of training. These basic characteristics of modern nursing are still active and help to define contemporary professional nursing. Up until the nineteenth century, most caring for the sick was done in the home, either by family members or untrained paid carers. In his biography of Florence Nightingale, Bostridge (2009) describes the impact of the Industrial Revolution, leading to a shift of population to cities, disruption of traditional family support networks, and overcrowded living conditions in which diseases spread easily. At the same time, changes in medicine, including the introduction of anaesthesia in 1846, made hospital care more worthwhile in the treatment of illness. Larger numbers of patients, receiving more complex treatments, created a new demand for personnel who would be present around the clock, and maintain clean, safe conditions for patients. The emergence of modern nursing is thus bound up with the expansion of institutional healthcare, primarily hospitals, and with modern medical science.

Status has been an issue for nurses ever since. Systematic education of nurses imposed moral standards, as well as standardized programmes of knowledge and skills. Nightingale herself, in the preface to her foundational text *Notes on Nursing*, disclaimed professional status as belonging to medicine, not to be confused with nursing (1860/1969, p. 3). Indeed, her text was aimed not at a cadre of full-time nurses, but at "every woman [who] must at some time or other of her life, become a nurse, i.e. have charge of somebody's health" (p. 4). Even later, in her role overseeing the St. Thomas' School of Nursing, founded in 1860, she remained ambivalent about how much medical knowledge should be included in the curriculum (Bostridge, 2009, p. 455). In the 1880s and early 1890s, Nightingale was a firm opponent of registration for nurses on the grounds that proposed entry by examination would exclude less well educated working class women who were needed to meet the growing demand for nurses. She also believed that a test of knowledge, rather than demonstration of skills and character in practice, undermined what was for her, the vocational essence of nursing. Some of the themes in this debate persist as fault lines in modern nursing identity, even though the battle over registration was settled in its favour long ago. Nurses in developed countries now see registration and legislated standards of licensure as markers of professional status, and of nursing as a distinct activity.

Nursing continues to meet a social need which has only grown over time. World Health Organization (2018) data shows increases in the absolute numbers of nurses around the world. In developed countries, however, this may disguise shifts in the distribution of nursing work among different levels of nurse. On the one hand, Registered Nurses (RN) are expected to take more of a problem-solving role, applying sophisticated knowledge to clinical questions and delegating Practical Nurses (PN) or nursing aides to carry out traditional nursing activities maintaining cleanliness and comfort; this requires fewer RNs in proportion to the overall nursing workforce. In the other direction, Advanced Practice Nurses, such as Nurse Practitioners (NP) with higher levels of education are able to work more autonomously, especially in primary care and remote settings, and carry their own caseloads of patients. In crude economic terms, RNs are more expensive than PNs, and NPs are cheaper than doctors. Shifts in workforce are influenced by a number of factors, but one of them from within nursing is the rise in educational standards for nursing. Nurses who study for a degree, the thinking goes, may not be best employed making beds when they could be telling someone else with less education to do it. I have introduced these historically contingent shifts which are happening in the present only to underline the point that nursing *is* historically contingent. Nursing as we know it will disappear when either the social need for organized caring goes away, or some as yet unimagined alternative to nursing appears to meet the need.

Institutions

One of the sociological factors against which modern nursing emerged was the increased importance of health care institutions, especially the hospital. There is no such thing as nursing, in the modern sense, without institutions, including: hospitals, regulatory bodies, schools of nursing (and the universities, colleges, or hospitals of which they are a part), public health clinics, healthcare organizations (whether privately or publicly funded), and non-governmental organizations. All formal nursing takes place through the prism of institutions. Caring may be rooted in prosocial human impulses, but for nurses it emerges in a dynamic interaction with institutional conditions. Individual responsibility is important, but it is shaped, facilitated, limited, and expressed within institutional boundaries. There is a dialectical relationship between individuals and institutions, which is made up of individuals. Philosophers Martha Nussbaum (2001) and Paul Ricoeur (1992) have both drawn attention to this aspect of contemporary life. Nussbaum says:

> The relationship between compassion and social institutions is and should be a two way street: compassionate individuals construct institutions that embody what they imagine; and institutions, in turn, influence the development of compassion in individuals.

> (p. 405)

What Nussbaum has in mind when she talks about institutions, however, is somewhat different to my sense. She appears to be thinking more broadly about institutions as the embodiment of democratic political values that both express and actively maintain a health, free society. When I am thinking of an institution on a smaller scale like an individual hospital, it is obvious that hospitals can, and do exist in all kinds of societies, including those that are highly repressive. But the point about the interrelationship between nursing and institution stands regardless of the scale of the institution. Institutional conditions are also invariably multiple, so that for example a nurse is part of a network including employer, clinical team, professional association, or union. Elements in the network exist for their own reasons and are not necessarily in harmony, so that a nurse often feels pulled in different directions as a feature of institutional life.

The French philosopher Ricoeur makes a comparable argument to Nussbaum, defining, " 'ethical intention' as *aiming at the 'good life' with and for others, in just institutions*" (p. 172, italics in original). For him too, he is thinking of institutions primarily as political arrangements: "By 'institution,' we are to understand here the structure of *living together* as this belongs to a historical community – people, nation, region, and so forth ..." (p. 194) but again the principles of living together in aggregates that go beyond the individual and persist over time apply as well to smaller scale institutions. He goes on to define an institution as "a structure irreducible to interpersonal relations and yet bound up with these" (p. 194). This is an important point to understand nursing, which does historically, ethically, and in practice place great value upon relationships and yet cannot be reduced to them.

If nursing has grown up with modern institutions for health care delivery, and is integral to them, nursing's position inside educational institutions is not so clear-cut. At the inception of modern nursing, nurse education was designed on an apprenticeship model, in which nurses would learn whatever theory was deemed necessary in short stints in the classroom, and spend most of their time learning by working under the supervision and direction of qualified nurses in practice settings. I received my training under this system at St Mary's Hospital in London in the 1980s. At that time, student nurses were paid (albeit low paid) members of the workforce, operating in a strict hierarchy visibly announced by stripes on student nurses' hats (or epaulettes, for male students). As a largely self-contained system, of which Nightingale would have approved, nursing took its place within the social ecology of hospitals and healthcare. The historic shift of nurse education into universities, however, first in the US, then in other developed countries (ironically the US still has a non-degree route to RN designation while other countries like the UK and Canada have gone all in on degree level education for all new RNs) introduced all kinds of questions about the disciplinary status of nursing. Where does nursing belong on campus? Neither pure science nor humanities, it does not fit into either of the two traditional groupings. Law, engineering, and medicine are all realms of applied knowledge, where higher education is closely linked to professional status, and yet nursing, while sharing all these characteristics, is not as well established in the academy. Other practice professions like social work and teaching are perhaps our closest neighbours in terms of status.

Is compassion the essence of nursing?

Nursing identity has been debated since Nightingale's day, and the move to post-secondary education has continued to provoke debate (not least because of the emergence of a new class of nursing academics). Nurses have often sought status, identity, and credibility through a moral claim to being a profession centred around caring and compassion (Gordon & Nelson, 2006). Caring and compassion, though of vital importance for nursing, should nonetheless be seen in the light of the perspectives of nature and history, discussed earlier. It is reasonable to see nursing as a formalized expression of basic affiliative drives that can take the forms of caring and compassion, but human beings remain creatures of mixed and conflicting impulses. A brief historical survey of modern professionalized nursing reveals fault lines and competing interests that continue to play out. Both underlying forces, nature and history, are necessary foundations for nursing but they bring with them tensions that are not easily resolvable. That is even before we get to the situation of the contemporary nurse who needs to be educated, often to degree standard, with an extensive base of scientific knowledge, the application of that knowledge, understanding and skills in performing delicate and complex, technical tasks, and the relational skills of listening attentively to others and responding to their needs in a timely, respectful, and useful way. All this is carried out within institutional environments that require various kinds of surveillance and reporting, that set boundaries and priorities that may or may not be consistent, either overtly or tacitly – and performed over and over, while fielding competing priorities in the moment, almost invariably in a situation of limited, possibly inadequate, resources.

Caring and compassion are vexed and various human potentialities. They are not an essence of nursing that would be released pristinely all the time if only the "system" would allow it, or if only we could weed out the "wrong" people who apply to be nurses for the "wrong" reasons. There is an extensive nursing literature about compassion in nursing, which increased sharply following the Francis Report in the UK in 2013 into a case of widespread neglect and mistreatment of patients at a British hospital (McCaffrey & McConnell, 2015). One of the findings of the report and much of the focus of debate in the media, was a concern with a perceived decline in compassion among nurses. To put it into context, there were 29 recommendations about nursing, out of a total of 290, and those 29 covered a wide range of topics from the role of the Royal College of Nursing, to education of support workers, and nursing leadership up to the national level. The recommendations that attracted the most attention, however, called for changes to bring about "… an increased focus in nurse training, education and professional development on the practical requirements of delivering compassionate care in addition to the theory" (Francis, 2013, p. 1539). These included "… an aptitude test to be taken by aspirant registered nurses prior to entering into the profession to explore the candidate's attitude towards caring, compassion and other necessary professional values" (Francis, 2013, p. 1540). There was an implied association between practical, hands-on nursing care and compassion, whereas:

> Most of those with whom the Inquiry had contact agreed that the increasingly technical demands of the role required degree-level training and education. However, they recognized that the progress made in this direction had sometimes been at the expense of exposure to personal experience of the basic tasks that all nurses should be able and willing to do.
>
> (Francis, 2013, p. 1515)

In between the hedges of "most of those …" and "however …" there is a striking lack of interest in what "technical demands" might actually entail. Although the evidence presented in the report was shocking and disturbing, it did not demonstrate any causal link between degree level education and bad care. It is not immediately apparent why technical expertise should be any less associated with compassion in any individual than doing basic tasks. Elsewhere in the report, far greater emphasis was given to systemic factors that had contributed to a collapse in standards of care, including a top down insistence on meeting – or appearing to meet – targets rather than focusing on actual patients. There were also problems of staffing shortages, bad management, and hostility towards nurses who did try to report bad care.

Empathy versus compassion

Nurses, as perceived bringers of compassion, seem to have become at times the focus for a broader current of anxiety about perceived loss of compassion and empathy in society, reflected in the appearance of a flurry of recent books, some advocating compassion, others empathy.[1] Empathy has its advocates. Howe (2013) states that, "Sympathy is me oriented; empathy is you oriented" (p. 12) and defines empathy as:

> ... meaning "into feeling" or "feeling into." The idea of getting "into" a feeling is particularly important, particularly when we see and *feel* the world from the other's point of view, attempt to understand it, and seek to convey that understanding as we relate with those around us.
>
> (p. 9)

For Howe, some of the value of empathy is that it contains both affective and cognitive components, the latter including the capacity to maintain distance, to feel what the other person is feeling yet still be aware it is their experience, not one's own. Another writer about empathy defines it as, "... *the art of stepping imaginatively into the shoes of another person, understanding their feelings and perspectives, and using that understanding as a guide to your actions*" [author's italics] (Krznaric, 2014, p. x). Howe mentions compassion incidentally as an outcome of empathy, whereas Krznaric is at greater pains not to mix them up:

> The Latin origin of the word *compassion* means "to suffer with another." This is different from empathy, which can include sharing the joys as well as their suffering. In addition, the emphasis in compassion is on affective connection with others – feeling their emotions – and does not usually include making a cognitive leap to understand how their beliefs, experiences, and views might be different from our own.
>
> (pp. 11–12)

Advocates for compassion, on the other hand, put it as the more important experience. Armstrong (2011), for example, in her book *Twelve Steps to a Compassionate Life* explains the origins of the word:

> ... "compassion" derives from the Latin *patiri* and the Greek *pathein*, meaning "to suffer, undergo or experience." So "*com*passion" means "to endure [something] *with* another person," to put ourselves in somebody else's shoes, to feel her pain as though it were our own, and to enter generously into his point of view.
>
> (p. 9)

She then goes on to include empathy as one of her twelve steps, even though her "put[ting] ourselves in somebody else's shoes" sound very like the common understanding of empathy. Gilbert (2009), a psychologist with a more scientific approach, offers: "Compassion can be defined in many ways, but its essence is a basic kindness, with a deep awareness of the suffering of oneself and of other living things, coupled with the wish and effort to relieve it" (p. xiii). In another of his works, aimed at a more academic audience, he notes that, "Compassion is a complex, multifaceted process" (Gilbert, 2005, p. 53) and provides a more discursive account:

> Compassionate relating emerges from complex interactions between motives to be concerned for and improve the well-being of others, and competencies to be sensitive to others' distress with sympathy for, and understanding of, their position – with a complex array of cognitive competencies. At the same time one must be able to tolerate distress in others and in self to avoid defensive withdrawal or over-control. Empathic abilities that may being with emotional resonance mature with cognitive abilities …; these abilities, allied with a non-condemning or non-shaming judgement, support motives for care … Compassion also involves abilities for gratitude, generosity and forgiveness.
>
> (Gilbert, 2005, pp. 52–53)

Note, inter alia, that empathy appears here as one of the constituent parts of compassion. While the complexity of this definition does bravely attempt to unpack a felt human experience, in its very thoroughness it is difficult to grasp. Compassion becomes a concatenation of motives, competencies, emotions, psychological traits, attitudes, values, and behaviours.

Paul Bloom wrote a book with the provocative title *Against Empathy*, subtitled *The Case for Rational Compassion* (2016). His argument is partly based on the belief that empathy has received too much attention as the necessary basis for all prosocial morality and behaviour. He points out that many of our good judgements about behaviour, such as paying taxes or putting our waste in the correct bins, do not at all involve any emotional fellow feeling with another person. His strongest argument against empathy as such is that it clouds judgement and can be destructively partial. Empathy is a response to an immediate stimulus and as such directs attention to the here and now at the expense of wider context, longer-term consequences, or alternative points of view. It is not a very good basis for making good judgements about the greater good, according to Bloom. He finds compassion prone to the same faults, though to a lesser degree. In his distinction between empathy and compassion, empathy involves soaking up others' distress, which can be harmful to the empathizer, whereas compassion includes a kind of stimulus from empathy but is much more outwardly directed through the wish to help others.

Bloom cautions against the partiality that can come with empathy or, to a lesser degree, compassion. If compassion is primarily an emotional experience then it would be counter-intuitive to also expect it to be under conscious control, to be applied correctly as it were, taking into account all other expectations bearing on a nurse's decisions and actions. Feelings can be strong motivators to action but can become like the lamppost in the old joke about the drunk looking for his keys under a streetlamp. "Is this where you lost them?" "No, but I can see better over here." One of the lapses in care mentioned in the Francis Report was the failure to leave a glass of water within reach of a patient who could lift a glass and drink, but not get out of bed to fetch it. It is emblematic because it is an example of the most basic and simplest part of nursing care and to neglect it, not just once in a moment of forgetfulness, but repeatedly as part of a bigger pattern, is appalling. To take this one example, however, it is not hard to construct a thought experiment in which compassion or lack thereof is not a decisive factor in whether or not the patient gets their water. A nurse, filled with compassion, but for a *different* patient, might pass by without noticing the glass left out of reach. His or her judgement might be clouded by an intense experience of concern for someone else, whose needs may or may not be as urgent or as easily addressed as the patient without water. Alternatively, another nurse, coldly rational, who can readily bring to mind the most basic scientific evidence of the need of the human organism for hydration, might notice the position of the glass of water, gather its significance, and move the glass without any particular feeling, in accordance with objective information and perhaps an adherence to deontological ethics.

There was an interesting debate about this point in the nursing literature between two prominent writers on theoretical and philosophical questions in nursing, John Paley and Gary Rolfe. Paley (2013), writing in response to the Francis Report findings, made the case that social psychology was far more useful in accounting for the disastrous neglect and poor care at the Mid Staffs Hospital Trust than a lack of compassion in training, education, or personality of nurses. Rolfe and Gardner (2014) responded that the psychological studies cited by Paley, whose subjects had been students in various settings in the US, could not be applied to the situation of trained nurses in a UK hospital. Explanations of why people might not notice seemingly obvious things in their environment, for Rolfe and Gardner, should not be used to explain away nurses failing to use basic skills, not to mention observe the ethical requirements of their profession. I come away from reading the debate finding value in arguments on both sides, yet seeing both as incomplete. Minimizing social psychology and institutional context makes it very difficult to see why a certain hospital did so poorly in the first place, or why one unit was singled out as especially bad (as it was in the Francis Report). Over-emphasis on the moral core of nurses points to a suspicion that this hospital and one of its units must have gone out of their way to hire the least compassionate nurses they could find. That does not make much sense, and lends strength to the argument for social psychology. On the other side of the balance, Rolfe and Gardner are right to point out the ethical responsibility of trained nurses and to hold to account variations of behaviour even under the pressure of difficult circumstances of short staffing and poor management. Whether or not compassion is the magic ingredient, however, is less certain and more difficult to demonstrate.

Nursing as a form of humanist practice

If nursing does stem from basic human drives, favouring affiliative drives, and is shaped historically and institutionally – and if culture is a process of human self-reflectiveness enacted in the world, then nursing is both natural and cultural but always centred on the human world. This is not to make wider anthropocentric claims, it is only reflecting the reality that nurses work with and for fellow humans.

From this observation, it is a short step to a consideration of humanism with regard to nursing (McCaffrey, 2019). Humanism is a tricky term, used in many ways, that may even conflict with each other. Humanism can refer to the Western tradition of Renaissance humanism, with connotations of high cultural cohesion and continuity (and possibly superiority), but also of a spirit of open-mindedness and intellectual curiosity about human life, found in the works of early modern thinkers such as Francis Bacon or Michel de Montaigne (Toulmin, 1990). Humanism, in contemporary usage in the UK, is shorthand for secular humanism, meaning atheism allied to a commitment to scientific reason as the only worthwhile path to knowledge. Personified, a human*ist* can be someone who identifies with one (or more) of these ideals, or simply someone who teaches and researches in the humanities for a living. Commonly for nurses, humanism is used as a convenient term to refer to the interpersonal side of nursing. Beyond this weaker kind of usage, however, humanism holds potential as a way of looking at nursing and bridging with the humanities.

Another view of humanism is to think of it more as practice than as a fixed tradition or set of precepts. Edward Said, a literary scholar, argued in a series of lectures towards the end of his life that humanism is best seen "as an ongoing practice and not as a possession" (Said, 2004, p. 6). He did not want to endorse cultural tradition like a monument, but preferred to see it as a rich and living resource, always changing in light of present needs and concerns. For him, humanist practice was all about critical engagement, whose "purpose is to make more things available to critical scrutiny as the product of human labour, human energies for emancipation and enlightenment, and, just as importantly, human misreadings and misinterpretations of the collective past and present" (Said, 2004, p. 22).

From a nursing standpoint, humanist practice was for Said critical, dynamic, and inclusive, facing outwards towards engagement with the other. Nursing as a humanist practice still entails a central focus on human relationships, on caring and compassion – as well as the "human labour" of evidence-based practice, employing thought, feeling, and action, in networks, ecologies, webs, patterns, structures of human belonging and activity. Nursing as a humanist practice draws on humanity's capacity for self-awareness laid out as human creation in forms of language, images, and objects, as expressions of what matters to us.

48   *What is nursing?*

Note

1 No one thinks much of sympathy with the honourable exception of the ethologist Frans
de Waal who has studied prosocial behaviours in non-human species.

> We don't know exactly how empathy translates into helping or comforting behav-
> ior, but it minimally requires orientation to the other. Empathy can be quite
> passive, reflecting mere sensitivity, whereas sympathy is outgoing, it expresses
> concern for others combined with an urge to ameliorate their situation. This is
> what the parable of the good Samaritan is all about.
>
> (de Waal, 2014, p. 143)

References

Armstrong, K. (2011). *Twelve steps to a compassionate life*. Toronto, ON, Canada: Vintage Canada.
Bloom, P. (2016). *Against empathy: The case for rational compassion*. New York, NY: Ecco.
Bostridge, M. (2009). *Florence Nightingale*. London, UK: Penguin.
de Waal, F. (2014). *The bonobo and the atheist: In search of humanism among the primates*. New York, NY: Norton.
Center on the Developing Child. (2007). *The impact of early adversity on child development* (In Brief). Retrieved from www.developingchild.harvard.edu.
Eriksson, K. (2002). Caring science in a new key. *Nursing Science Quarterly, 15*(1), 61–65.
Francis, R. (2013). *Report of the Mid Staffordshire NHS Foundation Trust public inquiry*. London, UK: The Stationery Office.
Gilbert, P. (2005). *Compassion: Conceptualisations, research and use in psychotherapy*. Hove, UK: Routledge.
Gilbert, P. (2009). *The compassionate mind: A new approach to life's challenges*. Oakland, CA: New Harbinger Publications.
Gordon, S., & Nelson, S. (2006). Moving beyond the virtue script in nursing: Creating a knowledge-based identity for nurses. In S. Nelson & S. Gordon (Eds.), *The complexities of care: Nursing reconsidered* (pp. 13–29). Ithaca, NY: Cornell University Press.
Gottlieb, L.N., & Gottlieb, B. (2007). The developmental/health framework within the McGill Model of Nursing: "Laws of nature" guiding whole person care. *Advances in Nursing Science, 30*(1), E43-E57.
Howe, D. (2013). *Empathy: What it is and why it matters*. London, UK: Palgrave Macmillan.
Krznaric, R. (2014). *Empathy: Why it matters and how to get it*. New York, NY: Perigee.
McCaffrey, G. (2019). A humanism for nursing? *Nursing Inquiry, 2019*, 26:e12281. https://doi.org/10.1111/nin.12281
McCaffrey, G., & McConnell, S. (2015). Compassion: A critical review of peer-reviewed nursing literature. *Journal of Clinical Nursing, 24*, 3006–3015. doi: 10.1111/jocn.12924
Midgley, M. (2010). *The solitary self: Darwin and the selfish gene*. London, UK: Routledge.
Nightingale, F. (1860/1969). *Notes on nursing: What it is and what it is not*. New York, NY: Dover.

Nurse. (n.d.). *Online etymology dictionary*. Retrieved from www.etymonline.com/word/ nurse

Nussbaum, M. (2001). *Upheavals of thought: The intelligence of emotions*. New York, NY: Cambridge University Press.

Paley, J. (2002). Caring as a slave morality: Nietzschean themes in nursing ethics. *Journal of Advanced Nursing, 40*(1), 25–35.

Paley J. (2013). Social psychology and the compassion deficit. *Nurse Education Today, 33*, 1451–1452.

Ricoeur P. (1992). *Oneself as another* (K. Blaney, Trans.). Chicago, IL: University of Chicago Press.

Rolfe, G., & Gardner, L.D. (2014), The Compassion Deficit. *Nursing Philosophy, 15*: 288–297. doi: 10.1111/nup.12068

Said, E. (2004). *Humanism and democratic criticism*. New York, NY: Columbia University Press.

Toulmin, S. (1990). *Cosmopolis: The hidden agenda of modernity*. Chicago, IL: University of Chicago Press.

World Health Organization. (2018). *Nursing and midwifery personnel: Data by country*. Retrieved from http://apps.who.int/gho/data/node.main.HWF1?lang=en&showonly=HWF

4 Epistemic differences in nursing

If nursing is a humanistic practice, in the ways I suggested at the end of the last chapter, that is far from concluding that humanism is at the end of a quest to find the essence of nursing. I am cautious about even introducing humanism because of its variant meanings; for some it means the world of the humanities linked to empathy, bypassing science and technology, while for others it is the epitome of rationalism and science. Ironically then, humanism could appear on either side of the supposed paradigm battles in nursing between the caring-relational and scientific-technical. Humanism-as-practice from Said's account appeals to me because it suggests a possible way of thinking with humanism that relates to nursing-as-practice, based upon a responsive, recursive, developing interchange with the materiality of the world. In this chapter I discuss polarized views about science that have often resulted in limited, unbalanced ways of thinking about nursing as well as noting some of the authors who have created nuanced ways of restoring balance. I propose another way of looking at nursing, making use of thinkers from the humanities, that recognizes the rich mixture of knowledge and practices that takes place in practice.

Evidence-based practice

Evidence-based practice has become the predominant way of talking about applying scientific evidence in nursing work. It offers guarantees to patients and to the society that is underwriting the profession of nursing that nurses' actions are derived from verifiable knowledge and carried out according to good judgement of fit to context. Despite suspicions that it brings about an algorithmic, technocratic approach to nursing that undercuts personal caring, evidence-based practice incorporates both clinician judgement and patient preference into its patterns of decision-making. Evidence-based practice is not the monolith it has sometimes been portrayed as, and as Lipscomb (2016) puts it in his introduction to a recent collection of papers discussing it from numerous angles, "when I am ill I want the team who care for me to incorporate evidence into decision making whenever sensible and feasible and, I trust, this incorporation will be both frequent and enabling" (p. 1).

Application of evidence, however, is more than a straightforward cognitive process of retrieval and rational decision-making, followed by precise, reproducible actions (Risjord, 2010). Modern nursing may rely on evidence-based practice, but it is not co-extensive with evidence-based practice; they do not share the same boundaries. Evidence-based practice implies an even-handed application of rationality in which the nurse exercises judgement in response to changing circumstances, where only "patient preference" has power of veto over the evidence. When it comes to everyday practice, however, it is probably not often that nurses stop to consciously retrieve evidence – though they should certainly know when and how to do so – because within the extensive field of familiar situations and actions of experienced nurses, evidence is part of the background against which they operate. The field of nursing activity has scientific evidence within it, but what matters most of the time, to nurse and to patient, is the concrete manifestation of nursing knowledge. Evidence, in the interaction with the patient, is deployed overtly at times, and at others it is present as the blood circulation of the nurse is present – necessary, but out of sight.

Science takes time

If evidence-based practice is in a sense concealed in practice, it is important that nurses have a good idea of how the evidence got there in the first place and what is entailed in different kinds of evidence. Examining the place of scientific knowledge in nursing education, in contrast to questions of interpersonal relating, helps to clarify the significance of science and to place it more clearly in juxtaposition to the humanities.

There is a basic difference in how we come to know things that is sometimes missed in debates about what should be foregrounded in nurse education. Much of what is valued as essential to nursing identity, such as compassion and relationality, stems from ordinary human functioning and is part of life. It forms part of the basic human repertoire, although as the mixed creatures we are, not necessarily in evidence all the time and mediated by many kinds of influences. Some influences are external, while others reside within the person. Personality differences have an effect, for example along the spectrum of introversion-extraversion. Introverts tend to be more comfortable relating in smaller groups, while extraverts relate more readily with strangers. An introvert nurse might gravitate towards a quieter setting with more opportunity for one-to-one dialogue whereas an extravert nurse might thrive in the constant stimulation of the emergency room, and either in their own way could be an excellent nurse. Human sociability and affiliative drives are also filtered through cultural expectations of what is appropriate and desirable, combined with contextual inhibitions or permissions in the immediate environment. Thus, interpersonal relating is already occurring, one way or another, and it cannot be taught to student nurses as if they are *tabula rasa* and not complex, enculturated people with their own patterns of relating. That does not mean, however, that interpersonal relating does not need to be articulated, shaped, and cultivated into a form of practice that is nursing. That is the work of mentorship and role modelling, using applied knowledge from the social sciences and the humanities. How nurse education is structured and presented itself has a role as one formative inflection of how developing nurses will come to relate to patients, and how they will manifest compassion and empathy.

By contrast, no one is born genetically primed to know that the heart has four chambers or that 120/70 mm Hg is a normal blood pressure. Primed for learning, yes, but not to know actual pieces of verifiable knowledge. The large scientific knowledge base for nursing in modern healthcare can only be learned one piece at a time, to paraphrase Johnny Cash. Pedagogy that focuses on processes, on synthesizing and analysing data, and on complex problem solving helps learner nurses to bring knowledge into lifelike, then actual situations of nursing judgement and decision-making. But like a jazz musician needing to practice her scales and know the repertoire before she can improvise with others, the basic pieces of knowledge have to be acquired. The same goes for technical skills, for example learning how to give an injection safely, knowing where to place the needle based on anatomical knowledge of muscles and nerves, knowing what is in the syringe, the what, why, how and how much of what that substance will do, or may do, inside a human body. As Benner observed in *From Novice to Expert* (1984), all of this over time becomes part of the flow of practice, much of it unnoticed or unremarked until an unexpected variation triggers a new response, a change of plan that moves the attention to a new central point of complex knowledge processing, decision-making, and action.

Learning facts and technical knowledge takes time and deliberate cognitive effort. Medical science continues to develop, prominently today in the field of genetics, with the microbiome coming up fast – bringing nursing's knowledge base along with it if nurses are going to be capable of functioning as necessary collaborators in the delivery of health care. As actual or potential patients, or increasingly as consumers, our expectations keep pace with scientific changes or even outrun them in ignorance of timelines of research and regulation. Nurses are often in the position of brokering expectations against realistic possibilities and need to have a good grasp of the actual contours of the possible.

The kind of learning that goes into the formation (Benner, 2011) of a skilled, highly competent nurse therefore requires a great expenditure of time and effort in learning, of facts and techniques, but also of rational synthesis and problem solving. Over-emphasis on qualities like compassion can obscure this reality, just as the sheer weight of scientific learning can suppress wider questions about the full formation of an effective nurse. An effective nurse does practice with great respect towards others, sensitivity towards their subjective experiences, thoughtful curiosity about parts of their lives that might have a bearing on the encounter, alertness to context, self-awareness, and proportional emotional engagement.

One reality, many points of view

One of the misconceptions that bedevils attempts to capture the mingled nature of nursing is an appeal to "multiple realities". It is a phrase I sometimes hear from graduate students trying to grapple with different points of view that look and sound irreconcilable. Paley (2016) traces a slide from its original usage as a term to describe different social worlds to "a rhetorical marker for philosophical relativism" (p. 137). Often I find students are not making a serious claim to ontological plurality, and it is used more as if it is an attempt to sum up the view inside a kaleidoscope. But it is a phrase I discourage because it does suggest we can all live in our own separate worlds, somehow getting by respecting each other's reality when in fact we have to contend and cooperate within one real world in its materiality.

There are not multiple realities, but it is part of the human condition that we constantly negotiate our interpretations of reality with others. We can utilize objective facts but they cannot deliver us from the burden and freedom of interpretation. Our interpretations are inflected by personality, moods, physical states (a TV ad in North America showing Danny DeVito as an angry man transformed back to his actual, young, taller, reasonable self once he eats a chocolate bar plays on this), circumstances, values, emotions, desires, aversions – and once we come up against someone else's interpretation, we make our own interpretation of that too. In the following section, I discuss the ideas of three thinkers who have grappled with the human necessity of living in the world as interpreting beings, mingling different kinds of knowledge and experience.

Thinkers of the mixed

The British philosopher Mary Midgley notes that our thoughts take shape out of the influence of our existing assumptions about the world. "Our visions – our ways of imagining the world – determine the direction of our thoughts ..." (2006, p. 2). We are in the middle of life, looking out on our own horizon, formed by collective and individual legacies, before we even start to puzzle out conceptual problems or seek scientific answers. Midgley's goal is not to relativize the findings of science, but to explore modern human experience in which we occupy different mental spaces and draw in different kinds of knowledge. Midgley seeks a unified account of experience, following the same direction we saw earlier in her account of mixed drives. She is not trying to paper over conflicts or to smooth away tensions, but to try to account in a more fulsome way for the mixed nature of human experience.

> We are evolved animals, working under difficulties from inside the system. We use a haphazard mix of faculties which are not fully unified, but which give us various different sorts of useful light, so we had better try to use them realistically.
>
> (p. 169)

Midgley uses the analogy of maps in an atlas to show how we readily make use of different kinds of knowledge in the course of everyday life. An atlas shows multiple maps of the same geographic space on successive pages; one might have coloured blocks that denote political boundaries, another blues, greens, and browns to illustrate lakes, valleys, and mountains, and a third symbols showing natural resources and economic activity. Anyone who is familiar with how an atlas works knows that these are variant ways of looking at the same area without worrying that they somehow contradict each other or that one map represents the ultimate view. Each map is an answer to a different question, "but all these questions are still about a single world, a world so large that it can be rightly described in all these different ways and many more" (Midgley, 2006, p. 113). This pluralistic way of thinking is how we should think about nursing. It cannot be reduced to either art or science in any traditional sense, nor does it need to be reinvented *sui generis* as "caring science" or "relational knowledge" because these are synthetic categories that merely add new possible ways of looking at the phenomenon, or new pages in the atlas.

Michel Serres is a French philosopher whose dense, poetic body of work often comes back to a vision of the mingled nature of human experience. Serres was a mathematician and naval engineering officer before becoming a philosopher, and his early love of mathematical objectivity and practical work constantly inflects his writing. Analysis of separate elements and then synthesis are for Serres components of human sense-making. He likens the former to the preparation of raw ingredients and the latter to cooking:

> Fire fuses many things together. The raw gives us tender simplicities, elementary freshness, the cooked invents coalescences. Conversely, analysis slices and dices raw; synthesis requires flame. As a result, the latter tends towards knowledge and culture, the former remains unrefined.
>
> (1985/2016, p. 168)

Nursing practice, done well, is cooked with skill, imagination, and sensitivity. It tends towards knowledge and culture transmitted through the speech and touch of a nurse. Serres restores empiricism, so often used as shorthand for scientific atomization, to sensory engagement with the multiplicity of the world: "Empiricism, both cook and cupbearer, knows more recipes than laws, for the latter apply to homogeneous states of affairs and the former to mixtures, so frequent as to be commonplace" (p. 228). Data, sensory input, and synthesis come together in events of practice. Another way of approaching a blended vision of practice is through the idea of interpretation.

Interpreting the mixture

Hans-Georg Gadamer was a twentieth century German philosopher of hermeneutics, or interpretation. However, he saw interpretation not simply as a cognitive activity that we may choose to bring to bear on a given work, but as a constitutive part of how we go through the world as human beings. We experience the world already in it, already using judgements, not entirely consciously, to shape our reception of each new experience. The task of hermeneutics for Gadamer was to take the naturally occurring process of interpretive understanding and to strive to make it more deliberate and to strengthen our interpretations in connection with the world around us. He thought that the primary way of doing this was through dialogue with others, on condition of remaining open to (though not necessarily persuaded by) other people's points of view. In his landmark work *Truth and Method* (1960/2004), he stated his intention as thinking through the kinds of knowledge we have that are not produced by scientific methods. He was not against science, but he directed his attention to our everyday mode of life in which we make sense of the world without reducing experience back to objective evidence. One of his basic points is that science, in fact, relies upon hermeneutic understanding. No scientist begins from a standing start in the middle of an experiment: he or she first chooses a direction, an object of interest and only then applies the tools of scientific method to specific questions. But the choice of direction comes from elsewhere, from a personal response to something within the whole possible field of attention we all have, which is historical, cultural, and personal. When an astrophysicist announces to the public that the latest picture of a distant galaxy from a space probe is exciting or awe-inspiring, the adjectives do not denote objective properties of the cosmos, but using them demonstrates Gadamer's point. There is no intrinsic quality of being exciting in a cloud of gas in space but such judgements and the motivations for making them betray the drivers of meaning and value, of interpretation, that infuse scientific research.

In his essay *Theory, Technology, Praxis* (1996) Gadamer applies his ideas to the world of medicine. He acknowledges the increasing pressure of technology to shape medical treatment and decision-making but argues that it only heightens the importance of human discernment and judgement. Using algorithmic methods in care pathways or computerized systems might reduce the sphere of autonomous decision-making, but they only move the line of tension between the technologically determined and the kind of human knowledge for which each patient and each clinical encounter present a new question. Philosophers of the interpretive, the mixed, and the plural, map out ways of thinking about nursing that bring us closer to the reality of nursing practice because they are, in Gadamer's words, "radically undogmatic" (2004, p. 350) and open to new experience.

Interpretation in practice

Interpretation, perspective taking, and mingled knowledges are not abstractions but show up in regular nursing practice. A lot of nursing work involves persuasion, bringing a patient round to what we believe to be the right interpretation of what needs doing at this moment, or at least the optimal interpretation under the circumstances – you should get out of bed; no, you shouldn't get out of bed. The recent rise of anti-vaccination beliefs around the world provides a forceful example of the role of persuasion. Vaccines are an instance in healthcare where the evidence is clear and evidence-based practice leaves no room for doubt about what ought to happen – for example, a child of the appropriate age ought to receive the MMR vaccine, for the benefit of both the individual child and the wider population. But confronted by a parent who believes that vaccines are harmful, a public health nurse has to wade into the muddy waters of conflicting interpretations of the world and of the work of persuasion. Evidence is a tool of persuasion but cannot do the job by itself. Health professions have adopted the terminology of "vaccine hesitant" (American Academy of Pediatrics, 2019) to describe parents whose first response is to refuse to have their child vaccinated. It is a careful choice of words, which refrains from being too judgemental and thus confrontational, and implicitly leaves the door open to the difficult work of persuasion. It grants to refusing parents the possibility that they are open to persuasion.

In knowing the necessary facts and in being able to recognize when persuasion is called for, nursing enjoins epistemic versatility, an ability to exercise modes of knowing about the world, weighing their force and limitations, and how they contribute together to a practical apperception of a situation. Writers in nursing have suggested various ways of engaging this versatility. Risjord (2010), for example, outlines a web, or network metaphor for nursing knowledge. Kim (2015) proposes an intricate multilayered model of nursing practice that is carefully structured, and in the introduction to her book she also cites a metaphor of nursing being like a tapestry (Gordon, 1997). It is a metaphor that evokes the intricate combination of threads that together form a whole, which is visible as nursing practice, but the image of a finished product of course leaves out the dynamism of nursing practice across time, the continual constitution and reconstitution of threads that create a new web across the space of each new location, or a new tapestry in a new design.

Networks of knowledge that start from questions arising in practice can coalesce around different kinds of knowledge, or make use of some maps more than others to borrow Midgley's atlas metaphor. There are practice questions that will foreground knowledge from the humanities in combination with scientific knowledge. Where culture becomes an important factor in care, for example, there may be a need to draw on knowledge of religious beliefs, rituals, and customs – not necessarily in the sense of the nurse knowing about a cultural tradition in general, but perhaps of knowing who to ask, who best to engage in dialogue, how to negotiate the significance of cultural factors for a patient and family within the usual goals of nursing care in a given setting. Attunement to cultural difference is not a singular skill but more like a bandwidth of abilities that encompasses a reflective capacity to have some sense of one's own assumptions in relation to others, an ability to ask good, sensitive questions to find out what matters for the situation, and an imaginative reach to hold in mind that people value different ends, and for a multitude of reasons.

At other times, historical knowledge can help to shed light on a question. I worked with a graduate student who was a labour and delivery nurse. She began to see more women choosing to deliver by caesarean section without a medical indication, and then became troubled by the judgemental attitude of some health professionals, including nurses, towards these women. Part of her subsequent work to better understand the trend for caesarean by choice was to trace the ways in which the sphere of women's choice had changed over the course of the twentieth century, politically, legally, in the workplace, and in health care. The historical framework helped to explain how the choice for caesarean even became possible – in addition to developments in medical technology making the procedure safer and more reliable. Interestingly, the literature revealed obstetricians, using evidence of risk and benefit, arguing both for and against caesarean by choice. Unlike the case of vaccinations, evidence-based practice led to something closer to stalemate, so that the question of how nurses should proceed in practice needed to draw on other types of knowledge, as well as the scientific evidence.

Much of nursing care is conducted in language. One of Gadamer's insights is that language is the medium of understanding, how we make sense of the world. He also emphasized conversation as a basic structure for understanding – we can understand more, and better, only when we can let ourselves be open to other, new points of view. Persuasion may be one mode of language that nurses use, but even when the goal is to get someone else to see something our way, part of the process of getting there might well be to listen first.

Interpreting "non-compliance"

At one time in my career, I worked with a psychiatric consultation liaison team in a large general hospital. Our purpose was to assess patients admitted with physical problems who also had, or were suspected of having, a mental health problem. I went to see a patient one day who, we were told in our referral, was "non-compliant", which is health care jargon for someone who does not unfailingly do what we want them to do. He was refusing, some days, to attend his physiotherapy sessions. After talking to him for a few minutes, he smiled and confided, "Sometimes I say no just because I can." He was fed up with the discomforts of hospital, the sleep deprivation and unappetizing food, the surrender of control over his body, what would be done to it, where and when it was expected to be, so he asserted a little piece of control, some days, by refusing to move. This is an illustration of Derrida's incisive neologism, "hostipitality" (2002, p. 358). Derrida derived it from the etymological tangle of the Latin words *hostis* and *hospes*, from which we get host, guest, and hostile, but it conveys beautifully the experience of the hospital patient, pulled between gratitude and resentment, relief and fear. Labelling behaviour as noncompliance is one interpretation of a patient speaking from the squeeze of hostipitality, another is to allow for mixed feelings, to listen to what them, without needing to let go of a rational estimation that the benefits of treatment outweigh the disadvantages.

Motivational interviewing as interpretation

Motivational interviewing (Miller & Rollnick, 2013) is a method of interviewing that began in the addictions field and has expanded widely in health care because it is predicated on the dynamic of persuasion but before that on the reality of interpretation. Ambivalence is treated as an expected part of preparing to change, and to be ambivalent is to see something from more than one angle, to weigh pros and cons. One step in motivational interviewing is to ask someone addicted to a substance or behaviour what they get out of it, on the basis that behaviour has purpose behind it, even if it has become – or always was – an ineffective way of achieving the purpose. When I have taken part in exercises designed to have student nurses try out motivational interviewing, they often find this step difficult; it goes against the grain for them to look for something good to say, even from a fictitious client, about taking street drugs. It also goes against the grain of human egocentricity to put aside one's own interpretation to ask directly for someone else's. This does not mean that the nurses are supposed to let go of what they know about the effects of addiction, the neuroscience of addiction, of developmental and attachment theory, or of social determinants of health in setting a general goal of better or worse outcome for this client – but to work in the world of interpretation is to work in the world of the possible. When patients know they are ill, want treatment, and can make reasonable judgements about having to endure some degree of stress, discomfort, or loss of function in order to arrive at some better state overall, then the task of interpretation and persuasion may not be obvious. Nurses have all kinds of unspoken arguments, not least from medical science and normative expectations, on their side. When suddenly one thing in the chain of interpretation breaks down – one too many hospital meals, being woken up at 5 a.m. to have blood taken, not recovering as quickly as expected (another kind of interpretation) – then restitutive persuasion is called for. Human beings are already interpreting agents; nurses are required to work with interpretability within certain constraints, affordances, resources, towards broadly defined goals consistent with ethical and professional values and what is possible.

Conclusion

Nursing is a mixed practice. As Risjord (2010) has argued, thinking in terms of paradigms of thought that are irreconcilable and set up to compete for primacy is an unhelpful way of thinking about nurses. Networks that move in relation to the demands of practice, whether in the moment of practice itself, or at a distance through the medium of research and scholarship, are both a more accurate and more helpful way of thinking about nursing. Mixing, however, is not relativist. On the contrary, it makes it all the more important to assess the value, the permissions, and the limits of forms of knowledge. My argument in this chapter is part of my effort to focus on the humanities, and to work out where they fit in. Following Midgley, the multiplicity of nursing makes room for modes of artistic expression, as well as philosophy and history, to create the fullest possible picture. Poetry, for example, evokes forces that move human beings to thought and action or condenses moments of intense experience into words. Artworks portray more than visual reproductions of objects but also experiences filled with sense that call upon peripheral vision, both literally and metaphorically, to describe. Literature stimulates imaginative empathy to follow accounts of others' inner states and motivations.

None of this means valuing humanities at the expense of science or ignoring what only science can do, but it does mean becoming more precise in how we make use of both science and the humanities in the mixture of nursing. In the next chapter, I look at interpretation in the light of recent developments in philosophy that attempt to bring a scientific, naturalist outlook into dialogue with interpretive ways of thinking.

References

American Academy of Pediatrics. (2019). *Immunizations: Vaccine hesitant parents.* Retrieved from www.aap.org/en-us/advocacy-and-policy/aap-health-initiatives/immu nizations/Pages/vaccine-hesitant-parents.aspx

Benner, P. (1984). *From novice to expert.* Menlo Park, CA: Addison-Wesley.

Benner, P. (2011). Formation in professional education: An examination of the relationship between theories of meaning and theories of the self. *Journal of Medicine and Philosophy, 36,* 342–353. doi: 10.1093/jmp/jhr030

Derrida, J. (2002). *Acts of religion.* New York, NY: Routledge.

Gadamer, H.G. (1996). *The enigma of health.* (J. Gaiger & N. Walker, Trans.). Stanford, CA: Stanford University Press.

Gadamer, H.G. (2004). *Truth and method.* (J. Weinsheimer & D.G. Marshall, Trans.). New York, NY: Continuum.

Gordon, S. (1997). *Life support: Three nurses on the front lines.* Boston, MA: Little, Brown and Company.

Kim, H.S. (2015). *The essence of nursing practice: Philosophy and perspective.* New York, NY: Springer.

Lipscomb, M. (Ed.) (2016). *Exploring evidence-based practice: Debates and challenges in nursing.* Abingdon, UK: Routledge.

Midgley, M. (2006). *Science and poetry.* Abingdon, UK: Routledge.

Miller, W.R., & Rollnick, S. (2013). *Motivational interviewing: Helping people change* (3rd ed.). New York, NY: Guilford Press.

Paley, J. (2016). *Phenomenology as qualitative research: A critical analysis of meaning attribution.* Abingdon, UK: Routledge.

Risjord, M. (2010). *Nursing knowledge: Science, practice, and philosophy.* Chichester, UK: Wiley-Blackwell.

Serres, M. (2016). *The five senses: A philosophy of mingled bodies.* (M. Sankey & P. Cowley, Trans.). London, UK: Bloomsbury.

5   Cognitive science and experience

Sciences and humanities have been separated since the end of the Renaissance, and ever since people have been trying to work out their proper relationship, their meaning and worth in relation to each other. C.P Snow, who was both a scientist and a novelist, famously named "two cultures" in 1959, arguing that literary intellectuals had a woefully unbalanced outlook in which scientific literacy hardly counted against familiarity with the literary canon. Our familiar phrase, "the art and science of nursing" is a distant echo of the division. However, the two cultures divide falls short when it comes to disciplines of practical application in professional spheres such as medicine, law, social work, or nursing. They do not fit neatly into either of Snow's two cultures. One of the puzzles for practice disciplines is to do justice to the world of experience, in which we live and practice, in interchange with the world of abstract principle and scientific knowledge.

What I want to do in this chapter is look at ways of bringing together scientific and philosophical ideas about human experience that make sense for nursing practice and help to define the scope of the humanities for nursing. I start with carnal hermeneutics, a recent development in philosophy that takes a close look at how we live in, and make our way around in the world through our bodies and senses. Then, from a starting point in neuroscience, I discuss the work of Antonio Damasio, who builds a model of human cognition all the way up from the cellular to the cultural. From there, I introduce enactivism, which is school of cognitive science that advances a highly situated account of human cognitive functioning. Taken together, these three strands of current thought give a perspective that is materially-based *and* cultural, that takes into account both the natural mechanisms that condition human life (and are important for the scientific basis of nursing) and the efflorescence of cultural forms in which we live our lives, constantly making discernments of value, meaning, and purpose. I follow through an example from mental health nursing to illustrate how these kinds of developments affect nursing. By highlighting the role of interpretation in nursing, I suggest that space of nursing must be scientifically informed, but culturally active, and thus requires circulation with the humanities.

Starting from where we are

British philosopher Galen Strawson takes a forthright stance towards experience. He declares himself as a philosophical naturalist who thinks, "concrete reality is wholly physical" (2018, p. 160). But unlike some philosophers of consciousness, who proceed from a naturalist foundation to a scepticism about ordinary, perceived experience, Strawson insists that experience is a basic fact of human knowing: "The existence of experience is a certainly known general fact about concrete reality" (p. 161). Strawson argues that knowledge about the mechanisms of perception does not dispel the reality of perceived experience. Even if I were to grant that since my perception as I write these words of making letters appear on a computer screen is only really an unreliable impression brought about by a cocktail of neurones and chemicals, I would still be stuck in the experience. Experience is where we live. Strawson's argument is worth noting because he is unusually comfortable in straightforwardly arguing at the same time for naturalism and experience. He opens a space for thinking with physical explanations of phenomena while accepting we have to start from where we are, in experience. This is the space I want to explore in the rest of this chapter.

Carnal hermeneutics

Hermeneutics, as discussed in previous chapters, is a philosophy of interpretation that since Heidegger has advanced the idea that human beings constantly, necessarily make sense of their environment. It happens so naturally that it simply becomes part of our being, of how we are in the world. We know what things mean to us without having to stop and think – though sometimes we should, and sometimes we do, stop and think. Hermeneutics started out as an interest in the interpretation of texts but in the latter part of the twentieth century extended its reach based on this basic sense of ourselves as interpreting beings. Hermeneutics substantiates how we understand ourselves in relation to others, in social worlds, and how shared, cultural networks of meaning transcend the merely subjective. The idea that health is more than the absence of illness, for example, is not an objective, verifiable fact, but it is a shared interpretation of human functioning that has been enormously powerful in how people have thought about health in the past 50 years and in shaping the scope of nursing.

In the last few years, some hermeneutic thinkers have taken a renewed interest in the physical or bodily aspect of ourselves as interpreting beings. Kearney (2011, 2015) noted the different ways in which we use the word "sense" to refer to our organs and feelings of perception, including touch, as our primal modes of contact with the world, as well as "making sense" to denote higher-level processing and valuation of direct experiences. In his analysis of touch, he links *touch* to *tactile* to *contact* to the *tact* in con*tact* and says that, "to learn to touch well is to learn to live well, that is, *tactfully*" (2015, p. 20). This has resonance for nurses, who are licensed to touch people, with their own bodies or via tools and instruments, and for whom each point of contact requires tact to achieve the best ends with the least degree of offence (McCaffrey, 2019). Tactful touching includes respect, proportionality, and technical skill.

Treanor (2015), another exponent of carnal hermeneutics, points out that the body in its materiality has been relatively neglected in post-modern thinking, in favour of attention to texts and language. He warns against overcompensating with a rush towards "scientism" and asserts "*both* the inescapable nature of our hermeneutic condition *and* its ineluctably carnal character" (p. 59). Treanor continues his argument by taking up what he calls "the new realists" who accept the existence of a world independent of human perception that can be accessed by science. As noted previously, hermeneutic philosophers like Gadamer were not opposed to science, but were interested in how we understand in the flow of experience. What is new, and what runs through Treanor's discussion is the hermeneutic engagement with science, and most especially advances in neuroscience and genetics that tell us something about who we are, as a species and as individuals, how we come by our being-in-the-world and how we make sense of the world.

In relation to nursing, carnal hermeneutics opens up an ecological field of interpretation in which nursing encounters with patients are always conducted by, through, towards, and in interaction with physical beings in physical spaces. This return to the physical includes communications in language that have up to now been the usual focus of hermeneutic attention to nursing, but connects them back to physiology and actual consequences.

Damasio: brain, body, culture

Antonio Damasio (2005, 2012, 2018) is a neuroscientist who avoids strong reductionist claims about consciousness or culture. His model of brain functioning has three features that make it useful for developing carnal hermeneutics along the lines of a revitalized new realism.

First, he builds his model from the cells up, tracing the complex human brain up through increasing complexity of multicellular organisms. Starting with individual cells, he describes aspects of cellular behaviour following the imperative of homeostasis, of maintaining cellular life within narrow ranges of temperature, seeking nutrition, and repulsing threats. His point is that multicellular organisms, to levels of incredible complexity, are made up of constituent parts which, from the outset are in interactive exchange with their environment, and with their neighbours, expressing valuation of what promotes flourishing and what does not. Carnal hermeneutics goes all the way down to the cell.

Damasio's second major argument is that the brain is part of the nervous system which is an evolved form of regulation. The brain alone makes no sense without a body with which it is in constant communication, tied into feedback loops along the nervous system. He posits that our sense of self is grounded in the way the brain maps the body, giving us our sense of physical presence in the world that is at once so obvious, so immediate and so tantalizingly difficult to catch hold of. The brain and mind are carnal.

The third aspect of Damasio's work that supports carnal hermeneutics is his emphasis on affective life as part of human functioning. Again, he places this in the context of evolutionary development, with affect as part of the self-regulatory, responsive, evaluative functioning of the organism keyed to seeking optimal conditions for flourishing. Feelings "… are first and foremost about the body … they offer us the *cognition of our visceral and musculoskeletal state* as it becomes affected by preorganized mechanisms and by the cognitive structures we have developed under their influence" (Damasio, 2005, p. 159).

One of the attractive features of Damasio's work, from a nursing point of view is that he does not valorize the substrate of brain tissue at the expense of experience. Although he argues for continuities in natural processes all the way through from the cellular to the cultural, he does not make the mistake of believing that the cultural is reducible to the underlying mechanism. Rather, he says, "Biology and culture are thoroughly interactive" (2012, p. 312). Because of human capacities for self-reflection, memory, symbolic formation, and collective meaning-making, cultural life still has to be worked out in its own terms and experience is still, inescapably, where we live, however it is produced.

Enactivism

Damasio, as a neuroscientist, starts from the brain and reaches towards social and cultural life. Enactivism is a school of cognitive science that starts out both with the brain and with experience and conceives of them as intertwined together. Enactivism is usually traced back to the work of Varela, Thompson, and Rosch (1991/2016), who set out to explain cognition not as the operation of the brain processing inputs and outputs on the model of a computer, but as an embodied, interdependent circularity between biological structures, cognitions, and social and cultural existence. To do this, they drew on findings from previous cognitive science, the Western phenomenological movement in philosophy, and the Buddhist Abhidharma tradition that carefully examined human interaction with the world from the point of view of how we experience it. In his introduction to the reissue of the work, Thompson summarizes the main principles of the enactive approach to cognition (2016, pp. xxvi–xvii). The body and nervous system, as parts of a larger system, are adaptive structures of sense-making in interaction with their environment. Cognition, in this view, is this sense-making that goes on in embodied action situated in a world that is "a relational domain enacted … through [the human] mode of coupling with the environment" (p. xxvii). It is an ecological view of humans as cognitive beings where human experience is a necessary part of the picture.

Enactivism (Varela, Thompson, & Rosch, 2016, p. lxvi) carries forward some of the recurrent themes in nursing theory, for example the importance of interrelationship, of person-environment interaction, of human action as contextual and enculturated, and brings them into a theoretical framework of cognition that is also biological and neural. Nursing authors and researchers, as we have seen, have made use of phenomenology in philosophy, with varying degrees of depth and plausibility, but motivated by the desire to report back on what we find in practice, and to reflect on those experiences with the goal of improving practice. Enactivism is one development in contemporary phenomenology, that makes use of findings from neuroscience to extend Husserl's original project of elaborating structures of consciousness (Gallagher, 2012). It is also a return to Merleau-Ponty's (1945/2012) work on embodiment, which drew on the empirical psychology of his day.

Enactivism is one theory of distributed cognition, meaning that cognition is not solely a property of the brain, sending signals out to the body to make it do things based on mental representations, but that cognition is an emergent property of brain in interaction with the body, and in turn with the outer world. "The enactivists suggest that not just the brain, not just the body with its different systems, not just the physical and social environment – but all of these together play important roles in cognition ..." (Gallagher, 2017, p. 47). Consequently, characteristics of the body and of social and material environments become significant to the event of cognition. One of these characteristics is the idea of affordance, of what becomes possible for cognition. Having two eyes and two hands, for example, affords human beings a range of possibilities in the world, which in turn help to shape neural functioning and mental life. Physiological affordance is not only a matter of bodily form but also influenced internally, for example, by hormones, or physical states such as fatigue and hunger. In turn, affective states are a component of cognition, themselves related to physical sensations as well as established patterns of coping in response to contingent external stimuli.

Beyond the individual, in the enactivist view, cognition is further extended through interaction with the environment. Environment here means both social involvement with other people and the physical world, natural or human-made. Social life entails normative expectations that exert a powerful influence on how we are in the world, on how each of us manifests as our particular self, processed through multiple dimensions of socially held values and interests, permission and prohibitions. Likewise, the material environment presents its affordances that enable us to act in the world while at the same time shaping and directing our scope of action (Malafouris, 2013). Smart phones are an obvious example of how this works, especially for those of us old enough to remember life without them. Smart phones are the main conduit for social media, portable and ubiquitous. They, with the apps they contain that lend them utility, have shaped how we communicate, not only in the sense of that they are a tool for exchanging spoken or written messages, but also in how we use language – compressed, abbreviated, punctuated with pictorial symbols; they have shaped how people walk around, bent over, looking down, slowing down; how we behave in public places, speaking loudly to unseen listeners. Cycles of moral panic can move rapidly through cyberspace, creating waves of physiological arousal in those who take notice, for or against, by like or dislike, in feedback loops spinning through brains, nervous systems, eyes, thumbs, and social networks, all mediated by electronic devices.

Enactivist theory gives a model of human cognition that is in line with integrative models of nursing practice. Nurses are deeply embedded in material and institutional environments that provide affordances for nurses-to-be-nurses as well as bringing them up against limits of what is physically feasible or legally, morally, professionally permissible. It is most obvious in highly technological environments such as intensive care units how nursing skill and knowledge enter the world through complex, finely tuned interactions between minds, bodies, machines, feelings, and data as well as culturally shaped rules, values, and ends. Any one of these elements may become the centre of attention at a given moment, but all operate together and skilled nurses navigate them not by a process of disembodied cognitive mastery but in an embodied flow of responsive attention. However, even for those nurses like myself who are used to less technologically rich situations like inpatient mental health units, the role of materiality is no less important. Malafouris (2013, p. 72) notes how spatial arrangements in a built environment support choice, perception, and problem solving while setting up biases as to what kinds of choices, perceptions, and solutions are more likely to be produced.

An example of this point came out when I was interviewing mental health nurses for my doctoral work about how they saw nurse-patient relationships in day-to-day practice (McCaffrey, 2014). One nurse commented that, "I see a lot more nursing from the desk" – a succinct spatial image for a style of nursing in which the nurse remains behind the desk of the unit, observing patients across a physical divide and making decisions about interventions based on visible behaviours without necessarily engaging with the patient's underlying thoughts and feelings. There is more to nursing culture on a hospital unit than its physical layout, of course, but the nurse's phrase – shorthand for a mode of behaviour she assumed to be recognizable to another nurse such as myself – is a clue to how there might be a feedback loop between a space designed to separate one group from another, enabling members of one group to observe the other from a fixed point and one mode of behaviour becoming normalized at the expense of other options.

Mental health – nursing bodies, brains, people ...

Mental health nursing is a good place to work through potential results of carnal hermeneutics, at the confluence of Damasio's cognitive science and enactivist ideas. Mental health nursing exemplifies the Cartesian divide between mind and body that continues to shape health care organization since it assumes a separate realm of the mental. Carnal hermeneutics provides ways to work back against the divide, without resorting to reductionist views of brain chemistry. That reductionist tendency shows up in mental health nursing, via the modern bias in psychiatry towards biochemical causation, in a phrase I have often heard nurses use when reporting on the status of a patient: "we are waiting for the drugs to work". While there is some clinical sense in this, when you know that an antidepressant for example usually takes at least four weeks to show its effects, there is also a sense of helplessness for both the patient and the nurse. The patient is reduced to a receptacle for brain chemicals, and the nurse to a passive onlooker waiting for some kind of sign emanating from within the brain. All of the person's inner and outer life becomes side-lined in this deadly phrase. The reality too, is that antidepressant treatment so far remains a highly approximate game, throwing chemicals, mostly serotonin, at a brain in which we know, at an aggregated level, they are involved in the production of mood states. However, the other side of enactivist thinking means it is no longer possible either, given developments in the neurosciences, to ignore the brain as if there is an autonomous plane of therapeutic relationship free from the flesh.

Negative plasticity and trauma

One of the developments in neuroscience, which is affecting how we think about treatment and care, is brain plasticity (Costandi, 2016). Brain plasticity refers to the development and functioning of the brain at the organic level of brain tissue in response to inner and outer stimuli. It has become part of current language in some areas of mental health, especially as related to early child development and addictions. There is a normative arc of brain development in childhood in which neurones proliferate and are then pruned down. The basic arc of proliferation and pruning happens anyway, but the shaping in individuals is greatly influenced by stimuli in the child's environment. Different areas of the brain develop at different times, with basic sensory processes developing very quickly in the first few months, and higher executive functioning beginning in the preschool years, not finally stopping until the age of about 25. The most significant external factor that influences brain development during those early years of peak plasticity is the presence of a consistent carer who provides, safety, continuity, and stimulation. The term that is used for healthy stimulation in early development is "serve and return" where the baby expresses something and elicits a response from the carer (Center on the Developing Child, 2017). The game of peek-a-boo is one example. As well as the plasticity of development in early life, there is a degree of plasticity of brain changes in response to stimuli throughout the lifespan. In other words, learning and experience leave traces in the brain, traces that can become long-term organic changes with repeated exposure, as in practicing a skill, or with violent exposure as in post-traumatic stress.

Plasticity does not imply an unrestricted programme of self-improvement. Agency too is an emergent, conditioned property of humans in relation with materiality – there is no controlling subject standing to one side directing the process, as if we are outside of our own brains and plasticity means we can mould it like a lump of wet clay. Neuroplasticity has its own limits within human development, even if the precise contours of those limits remain to be mapped. Much of the work of plasticity is completed during phases of early development, ending by around the age of 25. By that time, patterns of behaviour and personality traits have already been established that continue to influence how individuals make their way through the world (however one sees the share of genetic and environmental influence in early development). Additionally, social and cultural norms exert powerful influences. While neuro-plasticity is an important discovery and helps to understand how we can continue to learn new things throughout life, or how traumatic events can leave lasting effects, it is by no means a way back to the Enlightenment myth of the fully rational human agent.

Catherine Malabou (2008, 2012) is a philosopher who has turned her attention to the concept of plasticity, with a focus on what she calls destructive or negative plasticity. She is partly responding to a tendency for plasticity to be subsumed into narratives of self-realization, of endless improvement, and personal responsibility cut off from physical, social, cultural, or political environments. Her countermove is to include various kinds of trauma that affect the substance of the brain under the rubric of plasticity and to think about the presence and significance of destructive plasticity in personal identity. She is particularly interested in traumatic brain injury of a specific type, that has a cutting off affect from cognition, leaving in its wake a changed self, cold, indifferent, and unmotivated yet still able to think logically. One of the consequences of this kind of injury is that the victim cannot think his way out of it, he cannot register the injury as an event in his own continuing flow of identity.

Malabou's (2012) account of plasticity, however, remains more concerned with the grand traumatic event than the fine grain of everyday life and exchanges that we may surmise leave the lightest of traces on the brain. For nurses, we generally meet the patient once the trauma has always already happened, and we enter the patient's world in light of the trauma, moment by moment. Malabou acknowledges different kinds of trauma under the rubric of destructive plasticity, but from a clinical point of view she does not delineate clearly between the various types. One distinction in cause is between the rare disastrous accident involving direct damage to the brain tissue, and the external trauma of events that make their mark on the brain indirectly, through the body, via the emotions and assaults on meaning and security in the world. These are events of physical, emotional, and sexual abuse, of traumas from war, political violence, or natural disaster. The scope of trauma extends from the domestic and intimate, which has its own horrors, to the geopolitical. Nonetheless, Malabou is right to point out that trauma, pressed into the plastic brain, has the potential to profoundly affect people's lives.

Mental health – nursing histories

These excursions along the borders of neuroscience and philosophy open up ways to think about mental health nursing. Nursing the brain is well-nigh impossible; it is the organ that gives us the sense of everything but itself; our chemical treatments are approximate in target and effects. Despite our growing knowledge of the brain's workings, we still have to carry on as we have always done, nursing people as we encounter them in their actions and their words. One thing we can say is that the more we know about the workings of the brain, the less helpful or certainly accurate our diagnostic labels become as any kind of objective description; they are poor representations of a shifting mosaic of behaviours and thought patterns underlain by complex pathways in the brain, clusters of syndromes rather than discrete conditions (Bentall, 2010). Rethinking how we define mental disorders may be a way of incorporating the findings of neuroscience into clinical practices and relationships. Trauma informed care is becoming increasingly important to clinicians as a way of registering the effects of negative plasticity, to use Malabou's term, while developing ways to help patients in relation to their own lived situation.

When we think about trauma, we may be thinking about neglect or abuse in early childhood, which has left long lasting tracks of difficulty in relationships, and increased likelihood of addictions or mental illness in later life; or of events, whether singular or repeated, that have occurred later on in life and have disrupted what might otherwise have been a relatively untroubled course of life. These have different implications for care, in terms of the resources available to the person for reflection, comparison, and constructive coping. In either case, however, the medium of care must be the story, which is carried in the cells but lived in daily life, the experiential story that will be part revealed, part hidden in the psychiatric history. When we come to story and history, we are back in more familiar hermeneutic territory. Mental health nursing comes to include in its scope of attention personal story, clinical history, and what I will call capital-H history, or the big events that roll over individuals regardless of who they are, or their personal histories.

I recall a moment during a group session on a geriatric psychiatry unit when one woman talked about how she and her family had been expelled from the Sudetenland by Czechoslovakia after the end of World War II because they were German; another woman then shared her experience of being forcibly removed with her family from their home on the west coast of Canada and interned because they were Japanese-Canadian. Each of them recalled the weight limit of possessions they could take with them, one in kilograms, one in pounds. They were both experiencing depression and anxiety later in life when these things came back to them. If there was anything therapeutic about that moment, it was not in my noting the poignancy of their parallel experience, but of them recognizing themselves in another, each as victims of capital-H History crashing into their lives. But what we as clinicians had done was to create and care for the space of the group as a place of trust and exchange.

The restitution of story to history through the lasting reverberations of trauma has a further development in what is called intergenerational trauma. In the Canadian context, this has emerged in relation to indigenous people following the Truth and Reconciliation Commission [TRC] that reported in 2015. The focus of the TRC was the history in Canada of Indian Residential Schools, that were established as a programme of forced assimilation. In the words of Sir John A. MacDonald, Canada's most famous nineteenth century prime minister:

> ... Indian children should be withdrawn as much as possible from the parental influence, and the only way to do that would be to put them in

central training industrial schools where they will acquire the habits and modes of thought of white men.

(Quoted in Truth and Reconciliation Commission, 2015, p. 2)

It was a programme of cultural elimination in which children were removed from their families and their communities, forbidden to use their own languages, and taught to despise their culture. That was how the schools were supposed to work, but since they were poorly funded and badly supervised, they were also breeding grounds for physical abuse, sexual abuse, and disease. The programme started in 1880 and the last school did not close until 1996.

The concept of intergenerational trauma is that trauma, especially when experienced at the level of entire communities and cultural groups, affects later generations who did not directly experience the original source of trauma (Isobel, Goodyear, Furness, & Foster, 2018). Systemic, decades-long assaults on familial and cultural bonds of affiliation and identity have resulted in high rates of family breakdown, addictions, and suicide. Under these conditions, clinical history not only has to include the personal story, but also capital-H History. The destructive plasticity of trauma inhabits the confluence of History/history, it is bound with place, language, ceremony, narratives; therapeutic interventions need to be made of the same stuff. The role of the nurse is thus thoroughly hermeneutic, not narrowly confined to conventional health science.

Malabou (2008) posits a dialectic of biologic and experiential:

> … the transition from a purely biological entity to a mental entity takes place in the struggle of the one against the other, producing the truth of their relation [and] plasticity, rethought philosophically, could be the name of this *entre-deux*.
>
> (pp. 81–82)

Nursing practice is another name for the *entre-deux*, the new negotiation between biology, scientific knowledge, the lived history, and the suffering person.

Carnal hermeneutics opens up a new nursing standpoint which takes into account the technological and scientific aspects of nursing and puts them into play in such a way that carnality is not static and reductionist, but reveals indeterminacy, plasticity, and interpretability at the level of human concerns and relationships. Carnal hermeneutics brings together what nurses already know in practice about shuttling back and forth between objective and subjective, flesh and culture, history and story.

Conclusion

Over the course of the last three chapters, I have been attempting to engage with science and the humanities in the way that nurses in the moment of practice engage with them – drawing on knowledge interpretively, imaginatively, and creatively. It is my thesis that only by thinking about the humanities in relation to science, and not as a separate department, can we get the true measure of what the humanities bring to nursing and how to make the best use of the humanities for nursing. I have chosen in this chapter to lead with carnal hermeneutics, since it is a philosophical tradition of advocating for the humanities in a technocratic age, but to follow it to a point of confluence where it meets cognitive science. At this point of confluence, the world of practice becomes a subtle, intricate network of effects which are ultimately material effects, though known to us as our own experience. The popularity of phenomenology in nursing research has been heavily criticized (Paley, 2016), and indeed studies often provide not much more than nice-to-know impressions of a defined patch of experience. But, behind the phenomenological research endeavour is an imperative felt by many nurses to do justice to what their patients go through and to try to improve those elements in the health care environment that we can influence, not least the words and actions of nurses. In the substance of nursing practice, we cannot bypass either the materiality of our carnal being, nor the cultural layers of immediate experience. In the present context, advocating for the humanities, I emphasize the latter. Since we are always already leading lives in culture, it is incumbent upon nurses to become adept at discerning the demands of enculturated lives, as much as it is to be able to register the signs of hypovolemic shock. Becoming adept means going through the humanities, developing and fine tuning discernment among the stimuli of a material, carnal world.

References

Bentall, R.P. (2010). *Doctoring the mind: Why psychiatric treatments fail.* London, UK: Penguin.

Center on the Developing Child. (2017). *Serve and return.* Retrieved from https://devel opingchild.harvard.edu/science/key-concepts/serve-and-return/

Costandi, M. (2016). *Neuroplasticity.* Cambridge, MA: MIT Press.

Damasio, A. (2005). *Descartes' error: Emotion, reason, and the human brain.* New York, NY: Penguin.

Damasio, A. (2012). *Self comes to mind: Constructing the conscious brain.* New York, NY: Vintage.

Damasio, A. (2018). *The strange order of things: Life, feeling, and the making of cultures.* New York, NY: Pantheon.

Gadamer, H.G. (2004). *Truth and method* (J. Weinsheimer & D.G. Marshall, Trans.). New York, NY: Continuum.

Gallagher, S. (2012). *Phenomenology.* New York, NY: Palgrave Macmillan.

Gallagher, S. (2017). *Enactivist interventions: Rethinking the mind.* New York, NY: Oxford University Press.

Isobel, S., Goodyear, M., Furness, T., & Foster, K. (2018). Preventing intergenerational trauma transmission: A critical interpretive synthesis. *Journal of Clinical Nursing, 28,* 1100–1113. doi: 10.1111/jocn.14735

Kearney, R. (2011). Diacritical hermeneutics. *Journal of Applied Hermeneutics,* 2011. Article 1

Kearney, R. (2015). The wager of carnal hermeneutics. In R. Kearney & B. Treanor (Eds.), *Carnal hermeneutics* (pp. 15–56). New York, NY: Fordham University Press.

Kearney, R., & Treanor, B. (Eds.). (2015). *Carnal hermeneutics*. New York, NY: Fordham University Press.

Malabou, C. (2008). *What should we do with our brain?* (S. Rand, Trans.). New York, NY: Fordham University Press.

Malabou, C. (2012). *Ontology of the accident: An essay on destructive plasticity.* Cambridge, UK: Polity.

Malafouris, L. (2013). *How things shape the mind: A theory of material engagement.* Cambridge, MA: MIT Press.

McCaffrey, G. (2014). Host and guest: An applied hermeneutic study of mental health nurses' practices on inpatient units. *Nursing Inquiry, 21*, 238–245. doi: 10.1111/nin.12065

McCaffrey, G. (2019). Touching from a distance: Nursing and carnal hermeneutics. *Journal of Applied Hermeneutics, 2019*, 1–9. doi: https://doi.org/10.11575/jah.v0i0.68015.g51898

Merleau-Ponty, M. (2012). *Phenomenology of perception* (D.A. Landes, Trans.). New York, NY: Routledge.

Paley, J. (2016). *Phenomenology as qualitative research: A critical analysis of meaning attribution.* Abingdon, UK: Routledge.

Strawson, G. (2018). *Things that bother me: Death, freedom, the self, etc.* New York, NY: New York Review Books.

Thompson, E. (2016). Introduction to the revised edition. In F.J. Varela, E. Thompson, & E. Rosch (Ed.), *The embodied mind: Cognitive science and human experience* (rev. ed.; pp. xvii–xxxiii). Cambridge, MA: MIT Press.

Treanor, B. (2015). Mind the gap: The challenge of matter. In R. Kearney & B. Treanor (Eds.), *Carnal hermeneutics* (pp. 57–76). New York, NY: Fordham University Press.

Truth and Reconciliation Commission of Canada. (2015). *Honouring the truth, reconciling for the future: Summary of the final report of the Truth and Reconciliation Commission of Canada.* Ottawa, ON, Canada. Retrieved from www.trc.ca/assets/pdf/Executive_Summary_English_Web.pdf

Varela, F.J., Thompson, E., & Rosch, E. (2016). *The embodied mind: Cognitive science and human experience* (rev. ed.). Cambridge, MA: MIT Press.

6   Compassion and the *pharmakon* of the health humanities[1]

Drawing on previous traditions of medical humanities, teaching practices in nursing and other disciplines, and arts-based research, advocates for health humanities have staked out bold claims that the humanities can help to counter technical alienation in modern health care. There is a debated claim that health humanities help to foster empathy among students and practitioners in health care professions. In this chapter, I add to the debate using the concept of the *pharmakon* to propose that if the humanities do indeed have effects, then these must be effects of substance, and effects that are potentially dangerous as well as beneficial. I give examples of the humanities being turned to sinister ends, making deliberately selective use of their link to compassion. Finally, I propose that the goals of health humanities should include not only the stimulation of empathy or compassion, but also the recognition of tragic necessity.

Health humanities, empathy, and compassion

Empathy and compassion often appear among the goals of the health humanities, within the wider scope of cultivating more humane clinicians. In the disciplinary literatures, medicine has mostly latched on to empathy and nursing on to compassion, but they both seem to want them to mean a combination experience of accurate recognition of another's emotional state and then meaningful action in response. As I discussed in Chapter 3, there has been a lot of debate about the differences between the two and their relative value. It is not a purpose of the present chapter to decide between empathy and compassion, and I have followed the disciplinary bias of nursing by favouring the term compassion except where quoting other sources. It remains difficult to adequately capture in words the complex of emotions, thoughts, reasoning, bodily responses, decisions, and actions that comprise an event of empathy and/or compassion (and this only gets as far as the compassionate/empathetic actor, never mind what the intended recipient of the act perceives). Empathy and compassion are important, but they are phenomena of human relating that are complex, dynamic, and culturally and politically inflected.

Promoting empathy and compassion in health care practitioners is a topic of debate for the health humanities. Amongst recent texts about the health/medical humanities, Crawford, Brown, Baker, Tischler, and Abrams (2015) describe reading as "a tool for broadening empathy" (p. 56) and more widely argue that, "attention to literature and the arts can help to develop and nurture skills of observation, analysis, empathy and self-reflection" (p. 18). Cole, Carlin, and Carson (2015) make a very similar statement, with reflection repositioned as a means to cultivating empathy: "Medical humanities attempts to cultivate certain key virtues in and values of medicine, such as altruism, empathy, compassion, as well as certain qualities of mind by means of various reflective, interpretive, and reflexive practices" (p. 10). Jones, Wear, and Friedman (2014) take a more cautious attitude, questioning the easy chain of association that is set up in the literature from humanities, to humanism, to humane. However, while arguing against what they call "the instrumentalist justification" (p. 4) for the humanities, they replace it with "the intellectual practice of the humanities ... which encourages fearless questioning ... and refuses to accept the boundaries that science sets between biology and culture" (p. 4). While it is worth questioning the word association trail from humanities to humane, it could be that intellectual questioning is another kind of instrumentality. As an alternate strategy, in this chapter I attempt to deconstruct the instrumentality of humanities in healthcare through an exploration of the *pharmakon.*

Pharmakon – definition and Derrida

Pharmakon is a Greek word with multiple meanings, including "drug". It is the etymological root of the family of words to do with medications: pharmacology, pharmaceutical, pharmacist, and so on. Meanings of *pharmakon* also include "poison, charm, spell" (Barnhart, 2006, p. 785). Derrida made much use of its polyvalent meanings in his essay *Plato's Pharmacy* (1981), where he took up the use of the word in a work by Plato, comparing a written text to a *pharmakon.* Derrida's essay is about the ambivalent and fissiparous effects of writing compared to speech and for him the potency of the word lies in "the regular, ordered polysemy that has, through skewing, indetermination, or overdetermination, but without mistranslation, permitted the rendering of the same word by 'remedy,' 'recipe,' 'poison,' 'drug,' 'philter,' etc." (p. 71). He acknowledged the more literal sense of *pharmakon*, but even then to establish it as an agent of double meanings and mixed effects:

> One must indeed be aware of the fact that Plato is suspicious of the *pharmakon* in general, even in the case of drugs used exclusively for therapeutic ends, even when they are wielded with good intentions, and even when they are as such effective. There is no such thing as a harmless remedy. The *pharmakon* can never be simply beneficial.
>
> (p. 99)

Derrida, however, was much more interested in the linguistic play afforded by the use of the word in relation to language and emphasized its dynamic possibilities.

"The *pharmakon* is the movement, the locus, and the play: (the production of) difference. It is the differance of difference" (p. 127). He used two metaphors to underline the way in which *pharmakon* gets inside to have its effects, first as housebreaker: "Apprehended as a blend and an impurity, the *pharmakon* also acts like an aggressor or a housebreaker, threatening some internal impurity and security" (p. 128), then as liquid:

> ... the *pharmakon* always penetrates like a liquid; it is absorbed, drunk, introduced into the inside, which it first marks with the hardness of the type, soon to invade it and inundate it with its medicine, its brew, its drink, its potion, its poison.
>
> (p. 152)

Derrida was so taken up with the linguistic possibilities of *pharmakon*, however, that he insisted that it must be considered "a drug without substance" (p. 142), "as antisubstance itself: that which resists any philosopheme, indefinitely exceeding its bounds as nonidentity, nonessence, nonsubstance" (p. 70). For my purposes, I want to make use of the polysemic vitality of the *pharmakon*, while insisting on the *pharmakon* as substance.

Presented with a *pharmakon*, you have a choice whether or not to take it, but once taken it will change you, cell by cell. This is as true for compassion as it is for morphine, as true for reading a poem as it is for Prozac. In the previous chapter, I introduced the work of Damasio (2012), a neuroscientist who has advanced a framework for understanding consciousness that posits an idea of human beings as physically interpretive organisms. Human brains generate images in a constant stream that "are given saliency ... according to their value for the individual" (p. 76). Value is derived "from the original set of dispositions that orients our life regulation, as well as from the valuations that all images we have gradually acquired in our experience have been accorded" (p. 76). Another basic construct for Damasio is that of map making, whereby images are arranged into varied and deeply complex patterns of meaning. In other words, while we have original dispositions rooted in the cellular makeup of human beings and genetics, our horizon of selfhood is constantly modified in exchange with social and cultural worlds, to which Damasio, unlike other neuroscientists, accords great respect as the actual realm of human experience.

The idea I am suggesting, in the light of Damasio's account, is that we can think of the arts and humanities as mind–body altering substances. We, as human beings, go to immense lengths to alter our consciousness as we find it. To alter consciousness is to alter the body and vice versa. There is the obvious category of mind–body altering substances, such as alcohol, tobacco, LSD, or heroin, but also foodstuffs (think of comfort food), then the activities we perform to feel good, running and exercise of all kinds (the so-called runner's high), meditation, yoga, prayer, chanting, dressing up (or down), anything that causes sexual stimulation etc. If this seems to make humanities into more of a drug, then it also makes a drug into more of a *pharmakon*; we already have a sense from the placebo effect that a drug's efficacy can be an unstable compound of the drug and the idea of the drug.

Humanities as *pharmakon*

It is now possible to restate the arts-compassion link in another way, based on the arts as another kind of mind–body altering substance. Putting it more concretely, to posit that reading a novel, for example, is good for nursing students, is to claim it has a distant effect: the student who reads a novel in a nursing course today will be more likely to experience the neurobiological/subjective event of compassion when caring for a patient in six months' time.

George Steiner, in a polemic partly directed at Derrida, spelled out the physicality of art, in this case poetry, and its effects:

> As the act of the poet is met – and it is the full tenor and rites of this meeting which I would explore – as it enters the precincts, spatial and temporal, mental and physical, of our being, it brings with it a radical calling towards change. The waking, the enrichment, the complication, the darkening, the unsettling of sensibility and understanding which follow on our experience of art are incipient with action.
>
> (1989, p. 143)

Richard Kearney, a contemporary hermeneutic philosopher, discussed what he called "carnal interpretation" (2011, p. 8) whereby "Every carnal act and organ inscribes its own *imaginaire*" and "sensation is expression and expression sensation. Flesh is word and word flesh" (p. 8). Or as W.H. Auden put it more succinctly in his elegiac poem on the death of W.B. Yeats: "The words of a dead man/Are modified in the guts of the living" (Auden, 1939/2016).

One implication of taking the arts and humanities seriously as *pharmakon* is to see that, like pharmaceuticals, they may have beneficial effects, negative effects, or both, or none at all. A *pharmakon* is an interpretive substance since it alters perception, however subtly, and perception, or how a person sees the world, affects how she or he acts in the world. The arts and humanities would not matter, and there would be no reason to include them in curricula of health professions, unless they are a kind of *pharmakon*, an active substance.

Pharmaceuticals, as the most literal descendants of *pharmakon*, are set around with rituals of protection, authority, and propriety. Health care professionals are habitually shocked by the laity's disregard for correct ritual, which is called non-compliance. The reason for the ritual seriousness is obvious, that pharmaceuticals are known to have real effects on human beings, and their proper use is intended to maximize therapeutic effects and minimize harmful effects, through well-targeted delivery of specific agents at optimal doses: hence the "10 rights" of medication administration (Vera, 2012).

The meaning of the effects is, however, interpretable. Modern society has highly sophisticated structures of meaning to endorse what is or is not a desirable effect. While I was writing an earlier version of this chapter, the tennis player Maria Sharapova gave a press conference at which she admitted to testing positive to a performance enhancing drug called Meldonium (*Guardian*, 2016). It is a drug manufactured in Latvia for short-term treatment of ischemia by increasing blood flow. Sharapova said she had been taking it for ten years on the flimsy grounds that she has a family history of diabetes. What caught her out, however, was not that her pretext was medically questionable, but that there was a change in ritual and she missed it. Meldonium was added to the list of banned substances for tennis on 1 January 2016 (*Guardian*, 2016). To what degree she believed her own dubious rationale is irrelevant, because the structure of meaning for her sport shifted and what had been a matter of indifference (in terms of legality) became redefined as one of culpable harm.

The *pharmakon* of arts and humanities is likewise embedded in structures of meaning, and rituals of usage, because it too carries the potential for potent effects that may be judged desirable or harmful. To illustrate this point, I propose three strong counter examples to the uncomplicated assumption in the health humanities that exposure to works of creative imagination has positive effects. Poetry written by jihadists, and by Radovan Karadzic, the Bosnian Serb leader during the civil war in the 1990s, are examples of art expressly in support of destructive ideologies. However, they are also examples of art that makes appeal to compassion. The third example, of the Goethe Oak, is a brutally ironic example of the possibility that the arts and humanities may have absolutely no effect on ethical behaviour.

ISIS, war crime, Goethe Oak

> Father, I have travelled a long time among deserts and cities.
> It has been a long journey, Father, among valleys and mountains,
> So long that I have forgotten my tribe, my cousins, even humankind.

These are lines from a poem by Osama bin Laden (quoted in Haykel & Creswell, 2015, p. 6), in which he recounts his journeys from country to country through the persona of his young son, Hamza, and then explains in his own voice the reasons for their travails. First of these is the need to respond to "a world where the suffering of innocents, particularly Muslim innocents, is ignored and 'children are slaughtered like cattle'" (Haykel & Creswell, 2015, pp. 6–7). He then goes on to blame the "Zionists" (p. 7) for their attacks on Muslims, and Arab regimes for their failure to come to their defence. There is an unmistakable appeal to compassion in the poem, to recognize the sufferings of children, and then to take action to relieve their suffering. It is crucially, however, an absolutely selective compassion where the invitation to care for the suffering of one category of people is accompanied by murderous rage towards other kinds of people.

Haykel and Creswell (2015) put jihadist poetry into wider contexts of the popularity of poetry in parts of the Arab world, and its place as part of jihadi culture. They argued that poetry had a function in establishing the self-proclaimed ISIS Caliphate as "a fantasy world of fluctuating borders where anything can happen, including the recapture of past glories" (p. 9). While from the outside, it is easy to dismiss jihadi poetry as mere propaganda, it has a role within the structures of meaning by which Islamists seek to legitimize themselves, their values, and their actions.

My second example of the potentially dangerous effects of a humanities *pharmakon* is the work of Radovan Karadzic, who was found guilty of genocide at the International Court in the Hague in March 2016 (International Criminal Tribunal for the Former Yugoslavia [ICTY], 2016). Before the breakup of Yugoslavia and the outbreak of war, Karadzic was a psychiatrist and poet, at the crossroads of health care and humanities. His poetry, however, became an outlet for his Serb nationalist politics, which brought him to the leadership of the self-declared Bosnian Serb Republic in 1992 and to a new career of ethnic cleansing of Bosnian Croats and Muslims (BBC, 2014). Surdukowski, a doctoral candidate in law, wrote a paper for a legal journal before the start of his war crimes trial in 2009, arguing that the prosecution could "use Karadzic's texts and affectations to warrior poetry in the pretrial brief and in admitted evidence" (Surdukowski, 2005, p. 677). His article's title memorably begins with the question, "Is poetry a war crime?" (p. 673). If the examples cited in the article are anything to go by, Karadzic's poetry has little literary merit, but it is clearly intended to valorize a narrative of victimhood and heroic revenge:

When the time comes for gun barrels to speak,
For heroic days, valorous nights,
When a foreign army floods your country,
And wreaks havoc and causes damage in it,
That condition must be righted:
Then you roam your homeland on foot,
And your boots fight side by side with you.

(Cited in Surdukowski, 2005, p. 685)

Here again, however, the poetry has a different sense within a structure of meaning where historical memory, identity, and narrative poetic tradition are connected to a living cultural context. I do not know whether Karadzic's poetry ever was admitted as evidence into his trial; probably there was no shortage of other kinds of evidence that made it superfluous. The question in Surdukowski's title is meant seriously, however, acknowledging the power of poetry as incitement to action via impassioned response. W.B. Yeats interrogated himself on this same question when he asked rhetorically in a poem:

Did that play of mine send out
Certain men the English shot?

(1938/1982, p. 393)

It is the real possibility of incitement to action that makes a *pharmakon* of the humanities, and the moral indeterminacy of the action as such that holds out potential of both benefit and harm.

My third counter example of the link between humanities and compassion runs in a different direction. The Goethe Oak was an oak tree in central Germany, where Goethe reputedly wrote poetry while enamoured of a local noblewoman. Through its association with the great poet, it became a symbol of German humanism and civilization. In 1937, the Nazis built the Buchenwald concentration camp at the site, and they chose to build around the oak since to them it symbolized a link between German high culture and their own ideology. To inmates of the camp, however, it stood as a positive symbol of a German culture that preceded, and would survive the aberration of Nazism (Neumann, 2000, pp. 178–179). The Nazis' appropriation of the Goethe Oak had nothing to do with the content of his work, and was a grotesque reading of themselves as readers of Goethe, whereby "civilization" is apportioned by race and language, and not by the quality of relationships within a whole society. The symbol of the Goethe Oak standing in Buchenwald ruptures the assumption of a straight-forward link between humanities and humaneness. The examples above point to the potency of arts and humanities as substance, and as reminder of the possible differential effects and uses of the *pharmakon.*

Compassion, contingency, and Weil's necessity

My purpose in this chapter is not to discount a connection between the humanities and compassion, but to complicate it and counter the tendency to assume it runs automatically in one direction. I am convinced that the arts and humanities do have a place in nursing education and research and that there are different ways of looking at their relationship.

Not only is the *pharmakon* of the humanities a substance of polyvalent goals and effects, but the desired effect of compassion is itself unstable. Compassion is a fugitive experience, a human response that may or may not emerge in any given situation. A healthcare system, however, has to provide a threshold of consistent response, which includes technical competency and ought to include a flexible responsiveness, based on understanding of individual histories and needs. That is both an ethical imperative and a practical one since technical capability alone is not all there is to helping people improve or maintain health. Objectifying people does not help.

There are claims in the nursing literature on compassion that it is something like a steady state virtue humming in the background (Bradshaw, 2009; McCaffrey & McConnell, 2015). That, however, strays from definitions of compassion that agree it requires the stimulus of another's suffering. The former is more like a personal characteristic that makes a person more inclined towards compassionate action, and the latter is the moment of compassion appearing in response to a specific occurrence of suffering. One makes the other more likely to happen, but offers no guarantees. But if compassion is not completely reliable as a resource for healthcare providers, it does not therefore follow that we should forget about it, as one physician author suggested, in favour of purely external and observable behaviours that he labelled kindness (Faust, 2009). If compassion cannot be summoned to order, nor can it be denied when it does arise. Compassion may not be a necessary condition of providing high quality healthcare at any given moment, but it may deeply enhance an interaction and the ideal of compassion as a virtue may furnish a sustaining sense of meaning for the practitioner. In practice, however, compassion is a contingent event and the humanities are well suited to capturing the flickering of contingency in the midst of life.

At the same time, I have been making a case in this chapter for thinking of the humanities as part of the physical world, with real effects for embodied, enculturated human beings. Those effects are always implicated in human purposes and values. Even compassion can be wielded like a weapon when harnessed to destructive ends, it can be cut in half and turned against itself. I have purposely used extreme examples to make the point, but there are always questions of influence at play in cultural creation. The *pharmakon* of the health humanities invokes ambivalence and contingency, and its power stems from the tension between contingency and the necessity of its physicality. To find a different way of thinking about nursing, of flesh and blood interactions that entail suffering and response, I turn to a difficult, provocative writer called Simone Weil.

Simone Weil was a twentieth century French philosopher and mystic who died in 1943 at the age of 34. She was a deeply ethical thinker, who was preoccupied with what she called affliction by which she meant a state that went beyond physical suffering. Affliction attacks a life "in all its parts, social, psychological, and physical" (Weil, 1951/2001, p. 68). She emphasized the social, claiming "There is not really affliction unless there is social degradation or the fear of it in some form or another" (p. 68). She moved from involvement in left-wing politics to a deeply religious world view but maintained an unwavering concern with human suffering and the cultivation of human dignity. Her work is hard to summarize because it is scattered across essays, notebooks, and letters mostly gathered together and published after her death. She is a compelling writer, who conveys spiritual humility and utter conviction at the same time. Her work has been promoted by poets and writers including T.S. Eliot (1950/2002) and Susan Sontag, but even her admirers caution that her ideas are best taken "piecemeal" (Sontag, 1963). Sontag described the extremity of her personality, which shows through unfiltered in her writing, and called her, "one of the most uncompromising and troubling witnesses to the modern travail of the spirit" (Sontag, 1963).

Simone Weil belongs here, in a book about nursing and the humanities because of her psychological insights, her searching spirituality, and her grappling with the presence of affliction in human life. Against the grain of contemporary attitudes, her work directs attention back to the tragic limits in human affairs. As nurses, we can hope patients in many circumstances get better, and can move on from being patients. A good outcome for an individual, however, is different from expecting that patients will stop coming, or that even when many diseases have become preventable and curable, that diseases and injuries will stop happening, or that suffering as such will end. Nurses are in touch with necessity as Weil saw it, as the indifferent world of matter to which human beings, as everything else in the natural world, are subject. It may appear fatalistic but for Weil it was a matter of seeing clearly how things are, to see people in states of affliction so as to stand with them in seeking to ameliorate their suffering. It is a hard vision, and a profoundly humane one at the same time.

One of Weil's key terms was force, which she saw operating in human societies throughout history. In an essay about Homer's *Iliad*, which she called "the poem of force" she defined force as "that x that turns anybody who is subjected to it into a *thing*" (Weil, 1939/2005, p. 183, italics in original). Force in Weil's writings is not the same as necessity, but the two are related. Force is what happens when human beings, faced with the necessity of material existence, strive for security at the expense of others and create relationships of privilege and power. Weil linked force itself to its social presentation:

> prestige, from which force derives at least three-quarters of its strength, rests principally upon that marvellous indifference that the strong feel toward the weak, an indifference so contagious that it infects the very people who are the objects of it.
>
> (p. 199)

With the rise of authoritarian politics, led by cult-like leaders who thrive on fostering division and hatred, today it is not hard to see what Weil was talking about. But even in the realm of health care, large institutions, collective professional identities, and most of all technology also exert prestige which can hide the power dynamic Weil described.

Weil nonetheless found a redemptive aspect in the *Iliad* in rare "moments of grace" (p. 208) when Homer describes tenderness between husbands and wives, parents and children, or even mutual respect on the battlefield. "It is in this that the *Iliad* is absolutely unique, in this bitterness that proceeds from tenderness and that spreads over the whole human race, impartial as sunlight" (p. 208). The poem's bitterness:

> is the only justifiable bitterness, for it springs from the subjection of the human spirit to force, that is, in the last analysis, to matter. This subjection is the common lot, although each spirit will bear it differently, in proportion to its own virtue.
>
> (p. 211)

Subjection to matter, for Weil was "the hand of necessity" (p. 201) and she also called necessity "the relationship of things" (2001a, p. 43). Seeing the world as made up of things in relationship to each other is similar to Buddhist ideas of seeing the interconnection between things, so that one has greater insight into one's own ego-driven desires about how the world should that obscure what others might actually need. She said that, "Obedience is the only pure motive" but "obedience to necessity and not to force" (p. 43). Here there is a distinction between the necessity that is "the relationship of things" (p. 43) and force which is played out in human action. Force admits of exceptions to itself when people are able to connect to the even more fundamental power of necessity. Weil thus finds a link between the pressure of necessity and openings for grace and compassion. The *pharmakon* of the arts and humanities as substance reminds us of the same necessity, the same subjection to matter, even when it is tempting to escape into idealism. It can at its worst be used to incite resort to force, but it can otherwise bring us back to the necessity we all share, "the relationship of things" (p. 43) in which we live and die. Out of this necessity, at times, appears the contingent event of compassion.

Conclusion

Through seeing humanities in the metaphor of the *pharmakon*, and taking up Simone Weil's ideas about necessity, I have tried to arrive at a sense of the tragic that the scientific worldview so conspicuously lacks, because it enjoins us to wait for science to fix everything – including the problems science created – while life rushes onward regardless. If poetry can be likened to a drug, likewise a drug can be likened to poetry. Both are "modified in the guts of the living" (Auden, 2016). There remain vexed questions of how best to administer the *pharmakon* of the health humanities to students who have widely divergent degrees of receptivity or compliance. A didactic novel like *Still Alice* (Genova, 2009), for example, has obvious relevance to students learning about people with dementia. It carries traces of Weil's necessity, the brute materiality of a decaying brain lived out in the life of a fictional character. Empathy may result in action, in doing well by others (where for health professionals, "doing well" is a highly complex bundle of technical, emotional, cognitive, behavioural, and ethical activity), but what the humanities first teach is the fact of relationship, of contact with the raw shock of the other.

Note

1 A version of this chapter was first published in the *Journal of Applied Hermeneutics*, 2016. https://journalhosting.ucalgary.ca/index.php/jah/article/view/53292
Used with kind permission of the editor.

References

Auden, W.H. (2016). *In memory of W.B. Yeats*. Retrieved from www.poets.org/poetsorg/poem/memory-w-b-yeats
Barnhart, R. (Ed.). (2006). *Chambers dictionary of etymology*. New York, NY: Chambers.
BBC. (2014). *Profile: Radovan Karadzic*. Retrieved from www.bbc.com/news/world-europe-19960285

Bradshaw, A. (2009). Measuring nursing care and compassion: The McDonaldised nurse? *Journal of Medical Ethics, 35*, 465–468. doi: 10.1136/jme.2008.028530

Cole, T.R., Carlin, N.S., & Carson, R.A. (2015). *Medical humanities: An introduction.* New York, NY: Cambridge University Press.

Crawford, P., Brown, B., Baker, C., Tischler, V., & Abrams, B. (2015). *Health humanities.* Basingstoke, UK: Palgrave Macmillan.

Damasio, A. (2012). *Self comes to mind: Constructing the conscious brain.* New York, NY: Vintage.

Derrida, J. (1981). *Dissemination* (Trans. B. Johnson). Chicago, IL: University of Chicago Press.

Eliot, T.S. (2002). Preface. In S. Weil, *The need for roots* (Trans. A. Wills) pp. vii–xvi. London, UK: Routledge.

Faust, H.S. (2009). Kindness, not compassion, in healthcare. *Cambridge Quarterly of Healthcare Ethics, 18*(3), 287–299. doi: 10.1017/S0963180109090458

Genova, L. (2009). *Still Alice.* New York, NY: Gallery Books.

Guardian. (2016). *What is meldonium and why did Maria Sharapova take it?* Retrieved from www.theguardian.com/sport/2016/mar/08/meldonium-maria-sharapova-failed-drugs-test

Haykel, B., & Creswell, R. (2015). Battle lines: Want to understand the jihadis? Read their poetry. *The New Yorker*, 8 June 2015, retrieved from www.newyorker.com/magazine/2015/06/08/battle-lines-jihad-creswell-and-haykel

International Criminal Tribunal for the Former Yugoslavia [ICTY]. (2016). *Statement of the Office of the Prosecutor on the Conviction of Radovan Karadžić.* Retrieved from www.icty.org/en/press/statement-of-the-office-of-the-prosecutor-on-the-conviction-of-radovan-karadzic

Jones, T., Wear, D., & Friedman, L.D. (2014). The why, the what, and the how of the medical/health humanities. In T. Jones, D. Wear & L.D. Friedman (Eds.), *Health humanities reader* (pp. 1–6). New Brunswick, NJ: Rutgers University Press.

Kearney, R. (2011). What is diacritical hermeneutics? *Journal of Applied Hermeneutics, Article 1*, 1–14.

McCaffrey, G., & McConnell, S. (2015). Compassion: A critical review of peer-reviewed nursing literature. *Journal of Clinical Nursing, 24*, 3006–3015. doi: 10.1111/jocn.12924

Neumann, K. (2000). *Shifting memories: The Nazi past in the new Germany.* Ann Arbor, MI: The University of Michigan Press.

Sontag, S. (1963). Simone Weil. *New York Review of Books*, Feb. 1963. Retrieved from www.nybooks.com/articles/1963/02/01/simone-weil/

Steiner, G. (1989). *Real presences.* London, UK: Faber.

Surdukowski, J. (2005). Is poetry a war crime? Reckoning for Radovan Karadzic the poet-warrior. *Michigan Journal of International Law, 26*, 673–699.

Vera, M. (2012). *The 10 rights of drug administration.* Retrieved from http://nurseslabs.com/10-rs-rights-of-drug-administration/

Weil, S. (1951/2001). *Waiting for God* (E. Craufurd, Trans.). New York, NY: Perennial Classics.

Weil, S. (2001a). *Gravity and grace.* London, UK: Routledge.

Weil, S. (2005). *Simone Weil: An anthology.* (S. Miles, Ed.). London, UK: Penguin.

Yeats, W.B. (1982). *Collected poems.* London, UK: Macmillan.

7 Prose and poetry in nursing

Creative writing lives within the ecology of nursing knowledge: writing by nurses or about nurses; writing aimed at nurses, or communicating with a wider public, explaining, describing, evoking nurses' experiences, and giving insights into what it is like to be a nurse. Creative writing can carry emotional weight that is part of life among working with people undergoing times of vulnerability, sickness, dying, fear, relief, restoration, even joy – or boredom, nagging uncertainty, and pain dragging through every day. Creative writing restores the emotional weight that is conscientiously trimmed from conventional research reporting, that is treated as merely subjective, peripheral, and confounding next to the cool clarity of the numbers, or even of carefully cropped statements, units of meaning, arranged into tidy themes.

Human beings compulsively tell each other stories of how this was and how that went and why things turned out that way; we meet each other in stories, we bind our communities, sometimes heal, sometime wield them as a weapon against outsiders – but all that is to show that they are potent and we are caught up with stories as we are caught up with language. At times, statistics are just the thing to pull apart a badly made story, and at times a story is the best way of injecting life back into statistics.

Creative writing includes numerous forms, each with its own demands and its own way of bringing aspects of life into the light. In this chapter I discuss forms, for what they can communicate about nursing, and reveal about different parts of nursing life. I contrast the broad genres of prose and poetry, where prose follows conventional rules of grammar and syntax, building by sentences and paragraphs into larger units of meaning, and poetry is made up of smaller phases, which could be parts of a much larger whole, that are formed by sound and rhythm as well as meaning. Another distinction in how different forms serve different purposes and achieve different effects is between narrative and lyric. Narrative points to the function, either in prose or poetry, of storytelling that gets from A to B, if not necessarily always in a straight line. Lyric, which is often conflated with poetry, may have a narrative thread but does not depend on it, and often aims to illuminate moments of intense experience. In the latter parts of the chapter, I discuss the place of lyric in relation to nursing using the example of a short but potent poem.

Prose

Narrative medicine

Narrative as technique deployed for instrumental purposes constitutes a robust push back against automatic, algorithmic thinking and draws clinicians' attention back to the life of the patient, who has to live with illness, treatment, and their impacts. Narrative medicine has been developed by a physician, Rita Charon, as an intentional harnessing of narrative skills to clinical relationships. It is a specific kind of intervention, intended to complement the resources of medical science, as a way of deepening and sensitizing clinical communication to achieve optimal outcomes for each patient (Charon, 2006). To some extent, narrative medicine could be seen as one way of importing elements of established nursing practice such as presence and patient centred care into medicine. In return, the medical approach to narrative offers nurses a systematic, well-grounded framework for understanding how narrative is structured, so as to make more focused and effective use of narrative techniques. By analogy, narrative medicine follows basic medical logic: presenting problem = lack of empathy; diagnosis = failure to see illness as part of a person's life, not only as disease; treatment = elicit narrative – listen! Charon introduces technical skills of narrative analysis to then understand what is being carried in a story, using five categories of "frame, form, time, plot, and desire" (p. 114).

Narratives and nurses

Narrative is such a basic mode of human communication that it takes on a profusion of forms and functions. David Loy (2010), a Western Buddhist scholar, looks at narratives in a wide ranging, inclusive manner: "To be a person requires more than self-awareness: it involves some understanding of how I became who I am, and where I am going. Both are narrative" (p. 24). This sense of self unfolding over time emerges in nurses' work with patients, who move in and out of others' storied lives. Nurses carry in half-hidden forms, a responsibility to convey at least some unfolding parts of a person's story for the time they are alongside the person.

Where nursing work requires a 24-hour continuous presence, the day is necessarily divided into shifts. A side effect of shift work is that it sets a time horizon for the contact between a patient and each individual nurse, working in eight or twelve-hour blocks of time. Amongst everything going on for patients, they are often aware of the rhythms of handover, of changes in faces and personalities, as one cycle of hospital routines. For the nurses, handovers mark off the start and end to the working day (even if the day often gets prolonged) where a narrative of care has to be sounded out and passed along. Handovers can be telegraphic: lists of vital signs, symptoms, pain levels, behaviours, medications given or refused, bowels moved, fluids in and out … what changed, what did not change, what should have changed or changed unexpectedly … Narrative continuity, of the patient story, can get buried in information. Electronic health records accentuate the tendency – they are good for maintaining accurate and consistent lists but are designed to foster narrative-by-data.

Similar to Loy's claim about the importance of narrative to being a person, when I worked as an educator on an inpatient mental health unit for older adults, I used to simplify the significance of care planning across the time horizon of the shift down to "where from?" and "where to?" In other words, what has brought the patient here, what do they need from us to help them get to where they need to go to next? Note that Loy quietly says you need "*some* understanding" [italics added] (2010, p. 24) of the from and the to. It is not our job to "know the whole person" as holistic rhetoric sometimes has it, but to make good judgements about what we need to know to work with the patient to the best of our ability. Narrative is a good way of thinking how nurses and patients interact, how their very different stories for a while cross over, and they each become a character in the other's story. It is up to the nurse to try to make those stories mesh in a way that makes sense in the onward progress of the patient's life.

Nurse narratives

Recently, there have been several outstanding examples of narrative prose by nurses published in the UK. These are not applications of narrative technique in clinical work but works by writers who are or have been nurses, aimed at a general readership. The first was the acclaimed memoir by Christie Watson (2018) about her years of nursing practice. Her achievement is to portray in flowing prose the life of practice in its immediacy and in its contextual fullness, with ethical and emotional commitment and without sentimentality. The first chapter of her book describes her arriving at work and immediately receiving an emergency call as part of a resuscitation team. Watson packs a great amount of wide ranging information and ideas into this deceptively straightforward narrative event in a wonderful piece of writing.

She opens with a "tracking shot" as she walks into the hospital, telling us what she sees, weaving together impressions into a mosaic of an institution, a constellation she knows well, in which she has her place. Then running from her office in response to a resuscitation call, the tracking through the institution returns now with a sharply defined line, seen by the eyes of a nurse with her own goals, skills, imperatives. She introduces the reader in passing to the array of equipment at her disposal, to colleagues, conveying in brief observations a team rapidly assembled for this event – some with shared histories, some new arrivals – coalesced around a woman collapsed in the canteen; concern, care, getting to know the patient in a few well shaped moments. *Inter alia*, Watson tells the reader about heart attacks and how women do not always have the classic signs. Now she is going with the patient into the Accident and Emergency (A&E) department, into another subculture – there is a sudden backward look at the history of hospitals in London back to the Middle Ages, the emotional demands of caring for the sick down the centuries and then back into a busy modern hospital, looking for space in an overcrowded A&E. After further asides on the kind of nurses who work in A&E, on NHS staffing, and psychiatry liaison, the trolley and the patient and the nurse-narrator finally come to a stop, the patient comes into focus, with her chest pain, probably not a heart attack, that she is recently widowed and alone, her present in the light of her past, her story – and someone there to listen.

This is only chapter 1: a tour de force of fast-paced narrative, packed with descriptions of things, people, places, with facts and information, all of which weaves in and out of the narrative of *this* nurse on *this* day caring for *this* patient. Watson uses narrative to do what I have been theorizing about in this book, to convey the dynamic, interactive engagement of nurses with patients, bodies, minds, histories, institutions.

Molly Case (2019), still practicing as a cardiothoracic nurse, is another writer who has published a beautiful account of nursing practice, again mixing memoir, patient stories, technical knowledge, history, and family experience into a compelling, blended whole. Like Watson's, it is a work of prose narrative that does justice to what it is to be a nurse, that demolishes synthetic distinctions between objective and subjective, cool judgement and emotion, science and lived experience.

The third example is a book by Nathan Filer (2019) about schizophrenia. Filer is an ex-mental health nurse, who includes aspects of his experiences working with people diagnosed with schizophrenia. In his account he combines powerful accounts of patients and families' lives with careful consideration of the latest thinking about diagnoses, causes, and treatments for what is called schizophrenia. His focus is not on nursing as such, but his compassionate, intelligently sceptical approach to the topic – always returning to the central question of how best people can live and be helped to live with the effects of psychotic illness – could stand as an outline of what the best nursing care in mental health should look like.

When narratives break down

Sometimes narrative breaks down. Arthur Frank is a Canadian sociologist who has written about narrative from the patient's point of view, applying his academic knowledge and drawing on his own experience of cancer (2013). He has proposed a scheme of three different narrative types, the Restitution Narrative, the Chaos Narrative, and the Quest Narrative. Restitution narratives are, Frank says, our preferred type – stories in which one becomes ill, receives treatment, and is restored to health. In these stories, medical science is miraculous, doctors are wise, nurses are compassionate, and patients graduate successfully to health or perhaps to becoming "survivors". And after all, is some version of that not what we want for ourselves and those we love if we have to be ill at all? Quest narratives are more complex. In these, patients are less passive, there is a tragic recognition of suffering as part of life, and a kind of transformation of the experience of illness into an act of witness. Outcomes are less important than a true reflection of the depth of the experience, its losses and gains, the mourning it evokes, as well as the hoped-for relief. Chaos narratives, the last type, are accounts of being overcome by tragedy without hope of redemptive meaning-making. Chaos narrative, or as Frank calls it, "anti-narrative" (p. 98), is unreflective, unstructured, mired in the pain and panic of the moment, filled with hopelessness. The kind of narratives, in fact, that nurses may well be present to hear. To be able to sit and listen to someone for whom life feels undone, to feel sympathy without being absorbed into identification, to offer hope without trying to deny what you have heard is not easy. It is a moment of privilege and discomfort that is familiar to nurses, part of our personal narratives, and of the story of our profession. Chaos narrative extends the definition of narrative to include moments of incoherence and breakdown of structure.

Poetry and nursing

Poetry is a literary form, which can go to places beyond conventional narrative. Poetry at its best is speech under pressure – language that contends with the wildness of the world, with the unplanned and unwanted as well as with overflows of desire. Poetry has an affinity with nursing that is more than just the need in human culture for expression of intense feeling. Nursing is turned towards suffering, towards situations of pressure, and nurses often have to speak in such situations, to find something to say – with experience, judgement, and good grace, to find the right thing to say. From the side of poetry, Joseph Brodsky the Russian Nobel-prize winning poet, made this comment about W.H. Auden, whose work he greatly admired:

> It is the intonation with which one talks to the sick that cures. This poet went among the world's grave, often terminal cases not as a surgeon but as a nurse, and every patient knows that it's nurses and not incisions that eventually put one back on one's feet. It's the voice of a nurse, that is, of love, that one hears in the final speech of Alonso to Ferdinand in "The Sea and the Mirror":

> But should you fail to keep your kingdom
> And, like your father before you, come
> Where thought accuses and feeling mocks,
> Believe your pain …
>
> (Auden, 1944/2007, p. 417)

> Neither physician nor angel, not – least of all – your beloved or relative will say this at the moment of your final defeat: only a nurse or a poet, out of experience as well as out of love.
>
> (Brodsky, 1987, p. 372)

Narrative has become a significant way of organizing and communicating experience between patients and clinicians, or clinicians and public audiences. It appears in general clinical usage as well as a modality in psychotherapy, in research, and nurse education. We usually think of narrative as prose, even though it does not have to be in literature, where narrative is also a sub-genre of poetry. For advocates of narrative who want to find it, there can be fragmentary stories even in brief utterances, poetic or otherwise. Between poetry and prose, then, there are always exceptions but for now I want to concentrate on the lyric in contrast to prose narrative. In contemporary English usage, lyric is often what is meant by poetry in general (Jackson, 2012).

Poetry has an odd position in modern culture in the English speaking world, at times as approachable as a much loved pop song, at others as forbidding as *Paradise Lost*. It is a basic mode of speech, rhythmic and communal, at some moments and yet seemingly the preserve of academic specialists at others. There is in the nursing literature, a rich seam of writing of and about poetry, exploring its use in teaching, in research, and in clinical spaces but as with the humanities in general, it is a minority pursuit, full of potential that deserves much greater exposure.

An encouraging place to start is a special issue of the *Journal of Research in Nursing* in 2017 devoted to poetry (accessed at https://journals.sagepub.com/toc/jrnb/22/6-7). Macduff (2017) reviewed nursing's relationship with poetry historically, including Walt Whitman who served as a wound dresser in the American Civil War, and looked at nursing literature since 2001, continuing on from an earlier review (Hunter, 2002). He notes the uses of poetry by nurses, including as a therapeutic tool, as a means of provoking reflection for student nurses, or as a way of expressing findings in research. Rolfe (2017), using the broader brush of the adjectival form, notes the perfusion of poetic speech into nursing practice, alongside the factual and concrete, where "poetic communication aims to express what cannot clearly be described in words, through the evocation of images, sounds, feelings and memories" (p. 432). Breckenridge and Clark (2017), by contrast, zoom in on the strict tanka form from Japanese poetry in a shared, dialogic, practice of duoethnographic research. Their jointly authored poem is a work in which they reflect on their own practice experience, across contrasts of discipline, one an occupational therapist, one a nurse, and see it with fresh eyes in the light of each other's answering, interlinked verses. Their work demonstrates the way in which a formal discipline in poetic form can induce an obligation to bring feelings, thought, and experiences into condensed and direct words. By making use of the dialogic tradition in tanka poetry, they bring forth an interdisciplinary dialogue that would not otherwise surface in conventional, professionalized speech. Short and Grant (2016), describe a "hybrid pedagogy" (p. 60), in arguing that poetry is a language that cuts across normative social boundaries. They describe themselves as "hybrid academics" (p. 60) as teachers in mental health nursing who have also been mental health service users, and writers of academic prose as well as poetry. Poetic speech is not bound to institutional assumptions and can introduce a healthy scepticism towards our usual pedagogical and professional narratives – not because those modes of language do not serve necessary and important functions, but because they are not always commensurate with what people have to say.

The themes in recent nursing literature about poetry attest to the continuing vitality and value of exploring poetry and poetic language for nurses. While discussing the present and future relationship between poetry and nursing, authors note the alignment with the emergent health humanities movement (Macduff, 2017; Short & Grant, 2016). Poetry, as an art made of words, is the most literal example of a place where a distinctively nursing voice can contribute to the interdisciplinary conversation of health humanities.

Lyric poetry

There are moments in life when it does not make sense to expect narrative sense, when extremes of emotional or sensory experience force themselves into consciousness. This is the territory of lyric poetry. There are accounts in nursing literature of poetry being used in nurse education, for example to help mental health nursing students and clients find words for painful experiences and deep feelings (Raingruber, 2004). Poetry has also entered qualitative research as a way to present human experience (McCullis, 2013). Other than such instrumental uses of poetry, however, there has not been much consideration of lyric itself (McCaffrey, 2015). Lyric can refer to a form, a style, or a sensibility in poetry. It has come to be almost synonymous with poetry but has a long, changeable history back to its original meaning in Ancient Greece of songs accompanied by the lyre (Jackson, 2012). During the nineteenth century, it came to refer to short poems expressing subjective experience of mostly intense, brief emotion or sensation. Although the lyric form has come in for continued debate and critique, that remains a reasonable working definition. It can also refer to the lyric style used within a different genre of poem, such as epic. Edward Hirsch (2014), a poet himself, goes much further in his glossary of poetry. He stresses the lyric poem as "a space for personal feeling … against the grandeur of epic" (p. 356). This for Hirsch is what gives continuity to the whole history of lyric poetry, which he sees as a fundamental mode of using language. As such, it is not purely subjective, otherwise how could these brief arrangements of words still compel readers, and prompt intense emotional responses over centuries and across the world? Hirsch asserts, "The lyric poem immerses us in the original waters of consciousness, in the awareness, the aboriginal nature, of being itself" (p. 356).

One of the most famous descriptions of lyric poetry in English is William Wordsworth's (1802/1990) Preface to his collection of poetry with Samuel Taylor Coleridge, *Lyrical Ballads*, which has had a lasting influence on what we expect to find in lyric poems. He emphasized the element of raised emotion and outward expression in inner states, "to follow the fluxes and refluxes of the mind when agitated by the great and simple affections of our nature" (p. 871). But it is a subjectivity that is in the world of things and others, whose movements are not a sign of withdrawal but of close attention, "lively sensibility … enthusiasm and tenderness" (p. 877). There is an avoidance of abstractions in favour of description and sensory experience. Thus, subjective life and world are completely intermeshed and the poet "considers man [sic] and the objects that surround him as acting and re-acting upon each other, so as to produce an infinite complexity of pain and pleasure" (p. 880).

Though there is not much written about the lyric in health care itself, an exception is an article by Bleakley and Marshall (2012) arguing for the place of lyricism in medicine, using examples drawn from Homer's *Iliad* by way of a modern reworking of Homer by Alice Oswald. Oswald is a contemporary British poet, who makes superb use of the lyrical-in-the-epic in her long poem *Memorial* (2012). She names all of the dead soldiers referred to in Homer's *Iliad*, some with brief descriptions of how they died, and interspersed with Homer's own beautiful images from nature – lyrical moments it is easy to over-look in the onrushing drama of the *Iliad* itself. Oswald creates a distillate of loss and grief from the totality of war, showing and caring for the loss of each individual in the epic, one by one. Her work highlights the confluence of lyric poetry, and intense moments of nursing care.

Here is a free-standing lyric poem, without the tension Bleakley notes between epic, narrative context and lyrical moments that Oswald exploits so well. It is also a poem that is directly pertinent to nursing, beginning as it does in its title with one of the most ordinary and simple of nursing tasks.

I Carried Bedpans
I worked as an orderly at the hospital
without medicine and water.
I carried bedpans.
filled with pus, blood and feces.

I loved blood, pus and feces-
they were alive like life,
and there was less and less life around.

When the world was dying,
I was but two hands, handing
the wounded a bedpan.

(Świrszczyńska, 2016[1])

This brief poem is a lyric without the lyrical, in the sense of prettiness or con-solation. It is made up of a series of direct statements, from the speaker's point of view (which is that of the author, who served as a military nurse during the Warsaw Uprising in 1944 – when Poles fought to liberate their city from German occupation while the Red Army halted its advance and let the uprising be crushed). The first stanza is a series of bald statements of what the speaker did and where, but identifying it only as a nameless hospital – one with no food and water. In the second stanza, still in spare, direct speech, the speaker reveals a feeling she had, that she loved the body fluids she carried away in bedpans, and then states why in the first and only simile of the poem, because they were "like life". Between the last line of the second stanza and the first line of the third, she reveals some context, though still in terms that are general, or perhaps archetypal, rather than named, that life was shrinking and death was all around. In conclusion, she narrows the focus back to the bedpans carried in her two hands.

The bare, even blunt language, is similar to that of other Polish poets of the twentieth century such as Zbigniew Herbert and Wisława Szymborska, as is the directness of the gaze at a bitter reality. In this poem, however, the intensity of the attention towards one object, one task in the midst of a great disaster – alluded to but not named even as war, let alone the historical time and place – is what makes it so extraordinary.

Intense attention, without naming the context, lets the poem speak to carriers of bedpans in all times and all places. (It evokes for me a formative moment as a student nurse, feeling suddenly overwhelmed with sadness while carrying a bedpan in the semi-privacy of a sluice room in a London Hospital: I see the gentle Irishman whom I had nursed who had died a few days earlier.) To know that this is a poem of the Warsaw Uprising gives it tremendous emotional power, knowing that this necessary act of care is taking place amidst great destruction and heroism. None of that is stated in the poem itself, however, with the effect that it also transcends its moment in time and stands for actions that are done because they need to be done, even when circumstances appear hopeless. It is a poem of love and hope conveyed in the image of one of the most basic of all nursing actions.

It is worth comparing it to more familiar poetry written about war, which for English speaking readers, is predominantly the poetry of World War I. The best-known works were written by soldiers, like Wilfred Owen and John McCrae. Even where they focused on the pathos of war, on suffering and loss, it is from a soldier's-eye view. Świrszczyńska's poem is from a nurse's-eye view, cleaning up after the violence, where body fluids (I imagine them still warm) are the closest thing to life. There is nothing of the heroism of war, not even in the ironic or inverted forms of Wilfred Owen or Siegfried Sassoon.

This poem does what only lyric can do, conveying an excess of experience in a few words. It shows that lyric is more than just a style of poetry but is an attempt to capture in words a moment of being. Like the best lyric poetry, it "delivers on our spiritual lives precisely because it gives us the gift of intimacy and interiority, of privacy and participation" (Hirsch, 2014, p. 357). It is like Frank's chaos narrative, as a response to an extreme situation, but as poetry and not prose, it is not shackled to narrative demands. It was written in the 1970s, about 30 years after the experience, but it is "a masterpiece of lyric time, in which the presence of the poem can never be allowed to become a past" (Boland, 2016, p. 19). By concision and with enormous control of speech, it is vivid and immediate in description, of both palpable reality and the speaker's inner experience, yet its archetypal language creates a pathway to the reader's own experience. It stands as a moving memorial to an event in history, but it works beyond its testament to something that happened to someone else. As a word of lyric communication, it speaks to nurses who have known moments when time is suspended, when a moment of pure presence leaves an indelible memory; moments usually associated with extremes of experience, of dying, of profound mental disturbance, or of someone receiving catastrophic news.

Conclusion

Beyond the custom-bound genres of research reports and textbooks, there is much to be said by and about nurses that require different scopes of freedom, creativity, and expressiveness. I have looked at some of the possibilities in terms of genre with examples of prose and poetry. To conclude this discussion, I will end with the words of Molly Case, nurse and poet as well as prose-writer, who in this poem entitled *Spinal*, finds her mind drifting towards poetry while assisting with a delicate spinal block procedure. Seeing poetry in the crystal-clear drops of spinal fluid that emerge from the freshly inserted cannula, she decides:

> and I know that I can be both these things,
> poet and nurse,
> because if there's words there inside of you,
> then what's wrong with a bit of verse?

(Case, 2015, p. 45)

Note

1 Poem reproduced with kind permission of the translator, Piotr Florczyk and the poet's estate, translation published by Tavern Books, Portland, Oregon.

References

Auden, W.H. (2007). *Collected poems*. New York, NY: The Modern Library.

Bleakley, A., & Marshall, R.J. (2012). The embodiment of lyricism in medicine and Homer. *Medical Humanities, 38*, 50–54. doi: 10.1136/medhum-2011-010138

Boland, E. (2016). Introduction. In A. Świrszczyńska, *Building the barricade* (P. Florczyk, Trans.). Portland, OR: Tavern Books.

Breckenridge, J.P., & Clark, M.T. (2017). Two to tanka: Poetry as a duoethnographic method for exploring sensitive topics. *Journal of Research in Nursing, 22*(6–7), 451–462. doi: 10.1177/1744987117720824

Brodsky, J. (1987). *Less than zero: Selected essays*. New York, NY: Farrar Straus Giroux.

Case, M. (2015). *Underneath the roses where I remembered everything*. Portishead, UK: Burning Eye.

Case, M. (2019). *How to treat people: A nurse at work*. London, UK: Viking.

Charon, R. (2006). *Narrative medicine: Honoring the stories of illness*. New York, NY: Oxford University Press.

Filer, N. (2019). *The heartland: Finding and losing schizophrenia*. London, UK: Faber & Faber.

Frank, A.W. (2013). *The wounded storyteller: Body, illness and ethics* (2nd ed.). Chicago, IL: University of Chicago Press.

Hirsch, E. (2014). *A poet's glossary*. Boston, MA: Houghton Mifflin Harcourt.

Hunter, L.P. (2002). Poetry as an aesthetic expression for nursing: A review. *Journal of Advanced Nursing, 40*(2), 141–148.

Jackson, V. (2012). Lyric. In R. Greene (Ed.), *The Princeton encyclopedia of poetry and poetics* (4th ed.; pp. 826–834). Princeton, NJ: Princeton University Press.

Loy, D.R. (2010). *The world is made of stories*. Boston, MA: Wisdom.

Macduff, C. (2017). A brief historical review of poetry's place in nursing. *Journal of Research in Nursing, 22*(6–7), 436–448. doi: 10.1177/1744987117729724

McCaffrey, G. (2015). Lyric in healthcare. *The International Journal of Social, Political, and Community Agendas in the Arts, 10* (3), 1–8.

McCullis, D. (2013). Poetic inquiry and multidisciplinary qualitative research. *Journal of Poetry Therapy, 26*, 83–114.

Oswald, A. (2012). *Memorial*. London, UK: Faber and Faber.

Raingruber, B. (2004). Using poetry to discover and share significant meanings in child and adolescent mental health nursing. *Journal of Child and Adolescent Psychiatric Nursing, 17*, 13–20.

Rolfe, G. (2017). "I have nothing to say (and I am saying it)": The poetics of nursing. *Journal of Research in Nursing, 22*(6–7), 432–435. doi: 10.1177/1744987117727652

Short, N., & Grant, A. (2016). Poetry as hybrid pedagogy in mental health nurse education. *Nurse Education Today, 43*, 60–63.

Świrszczyńska, A. (2016). *Building the barricade* (P. Florczyk, Trans.). Portland, OR: Tavern Books.

Watson, C. (2018). *The language of kindness: A nurse's story*. London, UK: Chatto & Windus.

Wordsworth, W. (1990). *William Wordsworth: The poems volume one*. Harmondsworth, UK: Penguin.

8 Nursing, Buddhism, interdependence

Taking up the humanities creates an opening to look afresh at nursing from all kinds of angles. In my own doctoral work, I employed concepts from Buddhist thought to reconsider tensions in acute care mental health nursing; tensions between the therapeutic and the custodial, between "problems of living" in Phil Barker's (Barker & Buchanan-Barker, 2005, pp. 101–102) phrase, and neurochemistry, between relationship building and surveillance. In this chapter I draw on that earlier study to consider Buddhist thought in the context of its reception in modernity and how it holds ways of seeing the world that can illuminate the tangle of influences at play in nursing practice, with a focus on mental health.

Buddhism in the modern West

Buddhism in the modern West is strongly associated with meditation. Mindfulness meditation, which has become a branch of the global wellness industry (Poirier, 2016), is a secularized version of mostly Buddhist meditation techniques, first refashioned for people with chronic pain by John Kabat-Zinn (1990), who trained under a Korean Son (Zen) monk, Seung Sahn. Religious scholars, however, are fond of pointing out that in Asian societies where Buddhism has been a major, if not the predominant, religion for centuries it is far more about rituals and ceremonies than meditation, which is generally the preserve of monastics (Lopez, 2004). Nonetheless, despite an emphasis on meditation, Western Buddhists have imported other dimensions of Buddhist traditions and thought, adapting them in response to their own circumstances and preoccupations[1] (McMahan, 2008). For Westerners, Buddhism is rarely a religion one is brought up in, to be rebelled against in adolescence, but something one chooses – and being individualist, consumerist Westerners one can choose à la carte from a vast and varied tradition. Western Buddhism is a hybrid, as McMahan (2008, p. 19) argues, influenced by Western individualism, psychology, rationalism, and Romanticism but that does not make it illegitimate, just another new variation. The history of Buddhism is a history of adaptation as it spread across Asia, for example meeting with Daoism in China to form Chan (Zen) Buddhism. Extraordinary features of Western Buddhism include the rapidity of its reception and the accessibility of resources in modern translations drawn from the entirety of Buddhism's diverse 2,500 year history. This makes it conducive to the practice of "intercultural philosophy", which the religious scholar Morny Joy describes as "the practice of bringing one culture, language, or philosophy into another culture, language and religion/philosophy for the purposes of a clearer exposition of the relevant questions, contexts and topoi" (2011, p. xii). In this spirit, Buddhism is well worth exploring from the standpoint of nursing.

Buddhism and nursing

An interest from nurses in taking up Buddhism as a philosophical and theoretical resource is reflected in its appearance in nursing literature (see for example: Bruce, 2007; McCaffrey, Raffin-Bouchal, & Moules, 2012; Rich, 2007, 2010; Rodgers & Yen, 2002). As a body of thought that is increasingly being represented in Western discourses, it would be strange, in fact, if nursing were not to take it up. Taken as a philosophy, there is no reason to ignore Buddhism any more than other traditions that nurses have profitably brought to bear on disciplinary interests, from Aristotle to critical theory. The fact that Buddhism is a religion as well as a philosophy calls for some care in how it is considered, but it also furnishes opportunities for interdisciplinary study. At a time when scholars of religion and philosophy are exploring constructive dialogue between the two under the rubric of intercultural study (Joy, 2011) nurses bring the additional perspective of real-world application in a practice discipline.

When I first started to think about nursing in the light of Buddhist thought, I noticed several affinities between Buddhism and nursing. The Buddhist tradition begins with the question of suffering, with the existential fact of living a human life having to confront sickness, old age, and death (Smith & Novak, 2004). In our era of high-tech medicine, when even the phrase "old age" is considered tactless, and death is driven to the margins of everyday life, the very directness of this opening declaration in Buddhism speaks to nursing. Nurses, even compared with other health professionals, turn towards suffering and stand face-to-face with suffering unornamented; no amount of technological paraphernalia can ever quite fully get in the way. The next logical step in the Buddhist tradition is the call to compassion as a response to suffering (Nhat Hanh, 2008). Nurses are oriented towards compassion, however variously they enact it, by entering a profession of practical care for others. Another point of affinity is this emphasis on practice and not primarily in philosophizing or speculation (Rizzetto, 2005). For Buddhism as for nursing, this is not to say that there is no place for intellectual reflection, or that such reflection is not in itself a kind of practice, but it does mean that one is always accountable to the exigencies of everyday life, and in the case of nursing to those of clinical practice. Lastly, the Buddhist understanding of phenomena as interdependent (Nhat Hanh, 2006) speaks to the centrality of human relationships for nursing. This insight is reflected not only in relational nursing practice itself, but the ways in which practice takes place within complex networks of social organization, as discussed in earlier chapters. I will focus on this last affinity for the rest of this chapter.

Interdependence

Interdependence, or interconnectedness, has become one of the most widely adopted Buddhist concepts for Westerners, in part due to a receptivity that may not have existed even a few decades ago. Complexity science, ecology, and relational models of nursing all share a view of the world as dynamically interconnected. In Buddhism, the ontological claim that phenomena are ultimately not separate, and exist in relation to other phenomena goes back to the earliest sources. Originally, this vision of entanglement with the world was viewed as the very source of suffering, from which the Buddhist path showed the way to escape. In the later Mahayana tradition, it became associated with the concept of emptiness, which affords movement, growth, as well as decay to existence (Buswell & Lopez, 2014). Thich Nhat Hanh, a Vietnamese Zen monk and one of the leading interpreters of Buddhism for Westerners, has made what he terms "interbeing" central to his message of engaged Buddhism. He sees an ethical imperative in realizing, for example, how our food is made up of the land required for its cultivation, the labour of those who produce it, and all the environmental and human conditions that go into its appearance on our plates.

> Our happiness is made of the happiness of others, and our suffering is made from the suffering of others. So the understanding of impermanence, non-self, and interbeing inspires us to do everything we can to relieve suffering and bring joy and happiness to our everyday life.
>
> (Nhat Han, 2008, p. 266)

The Buddhist claim that all things, including the self, are co-dependent and impermanent gives rise to an understanding of how it is to be in the world, and to an exploration of the implications of that position. There is, in addition, a recognition in Buddhist thought of a tension between the philosophical argument that things are not ultimately separate from each other and the everyday experience that they (and we) certainly *seem* separate. It is from this tension that the emphasis on the cultivation of awareness springs, to try to bring one's immediate experience of the world more into line with underlying interconnectedness. Bernard Faure, in a discussion of Buddhist philosophy notes that, "The Middle Way [between no-self and sense of self] underlines the paradoxical nature of reality: It is a complex truth that cannot be reduced to any single formulation or any single term" (2004, p. 136). When it comes to practicing with interconnection, saying it does not make it so. In mental health nursing, however, it might point to the difference between treating a DSM-V diagnosis of depression as a finished statement about an individual whose brain chemistry is abnormal causing low mood, or a beginning insight into a person whose life is afflicted with low mood, brought about in a multi-layered experience of thoughts, feelings, personal history, social situation, and indeed neurochemical and genetic makeup. Interdependence comes back to one of the themes of this book which is the difficulty of representing nursing in its full complexity. In the following sections, I consider aspects of mental health nursing in the light of the concept of interdependence.

Mental health histories

On an evening shift on an adult acute mental health unit, I made the mistake of trying to talk to a patient about his anxiety. My problem was not that it was a bad idea, or that he did not think it might be helpful, but that I tried to do so at a moment during the shift when I was enacting two histories at once. While other nurses were on break, I had to sit at the front desk and monitor who wanted to leave or enter the unit, remotely unlocking the door as required. Not a demanding or difficult task in the routine of the unit, but as it turned out even a few comings and goings were enough to disrupt my well-meaning attempt to concentrate my attention on a therapeutic conversation.

Mental health nursing as a sub-discipline has two major streams flowing into it from the past, nursing of course, and the role of asylum attendant (O'Brien, 2001). Trying to have a joined-up conversation with a patient while taking care of the door meant trying to fulfil what I saw as my nursing role, as well as that of attendant. These two broad traditions are at play in inpatient mental health nursing (less so in community settings, though the locked door can still be represented by some form of compulsory treatment order). These two, however, are only the start of the tangle of forces at play in how nurses practice. The different histories that are in play within mental health units include confinement (locked door, formal patients under the Mental Health Act, orderly role); medicalized psychiatry (DSM taxonomy, assumption of chemical causes); medical power (control of admission, discharge, and final decisions about treatment); behavourism (giving and taking away privileges); psychotherapy (separated time to talk to patients individually or in groups); productive everyday activity (occupational and recreational therapies). Further still, if these are histories intrinsic to the workings of a mental health unit specifically, there are also less specific extrinsic histories at work that include the evolution of government funded healthcare, business management, and trade unionism.

Considering all this through the lens of interdependence does more than just say it is complicated. If the interconnectedness of things puts into question the idea of a fixed separate self, since the self is made up of other elements, then mental health nurses are made up of all these different influences. There is no essential self, standing apart to pick and choose among approaches to mental health nursing. As in my experience with the door, they occur at the same time or sequentially, smoothly or in conflict, partly in response to individual philosophies of care, but also on the back of circumstances as they arise. Therapeutic conversation one moment, giving a patient an injection against his will the next. Mental health nurses, to paraphrase Whitman, contain multitudes.

If one over-identifies with any one of these historical strands, the temptation is to desire that the unit as such be reconfigured after one's own image. To do so without being cognizant of the flux of historical narratives can end up in moral exhortation for one's own satisfaction. It is important to note too, however, that none of these histories owns the mental health unit, even though there are real power differentials. There is no final master narrative that controls the historical development of mental health units and all its histories deserve to be articulated and considered.

Causes and conditions/stories

One of the fundamental stories in Buddhism is that there is no fixed, permanent self. If this is true, then we need to hear how it can be that we feel as if there must be a self, that for better or worse we keep on being who we are. The answer according to Buddhist philosophy has to do with dependent origination, the idea as Thich Nhat Hanh put it, that "this is because that is" (2006, p. 82). A phrase related to dependent origination that often occurs in Buddhist sources is "causes and conditions" (Buswell & Lopez, 2014, p. 348), referring to the impossibly complex intertwined circumstances that brought about myself, in this moment, writing these words or you, in another moment reading them. In one possible translation of an ancient text, two co-translators rendered a Sanskrit word for causes and conditions as story (Nishijima & Cross, 2006, p. 179). The Buddhist tradition suggests that the problem with this constituted sense of self, or story of ourselves, is not that we have it, but that we identify with it so completely.

The causes and conditions of an individual self, in contemporary terms, would have to include genetic inheritance, early childhood experience, cultural environment including factors like ethnicity, language, religion, and economic status as well as a dense, evolving tangle of choices, preferences, and experience throughout life. When we are asked to account for ourselves, or more usually, some aspect of ourselves ("why did you become a nurse?" or "how long have you been feeling depressed?"), we do not, and cannot retrieve the whole mass of causes and conditions, we tell a story that is selective and shaped. Part of the Buddhist understanding of no-self, then, is that paradoxically there is too much self, it always exceeds our grasp, we can never know the whole story. At the same time there is no *primus inter pares* among causes and conditions, no separate element by which to select one, because they are never independent of each other. When it comes to ways of dissecting a self, whether for example by neuroscience or psychodynamics, any given account may be persuasive in its own terms and helpful provisionally, but each account is caught in the currents of causes and conditions and thereby changed at the moment of its knowing.

The self is not solid and unitary, yet impossibly multiple and tightly compacted. Understanding self as the result of causes and conditions, which we comprehend as stories works in two directions. In one way, we are bound to see ourselves according to our experience and hence to expect more of the same and in so doing we perpetuate the sense of a solid self, which may or may not serve to help us live in the world satisfactorily. At the same time, we are always in a story that is still being told, the bundle of causes and conditions, though tight is not fixed.

It is a familiar idea that nurses should try to find out about the patient's story, to put their presenting problem into the wider context of their lives, to locate the moment of the nursing encounter in a temporal flow of what has happened, and what might, or should happen next. Seeing the story as densely interconnected elements might have a number of effects. One is to enjoin some humility about the limits of what we can claim to know about anyone and another is to expect some acuity of judgement about what matters most at each encounter. There is a realism to accepting the difficulty of disentangling story lines in such a way as to help patients rearrange them to carry on living more satisfactorily for themselves, but also scope for actual therapeutic movement in doing so.

Labels

Buddhist tradition, in positing interdependence, also stresses the struggle ever to experience ourselves as not separate. Meditative practice steps into this space of seeing and not seeing, of wanting and not wanting to find that we are interconnected with each other and with our world. The place of practice is a place of recognition of the profundity of the sense of separateness, which never goes away. Practicing, whether with mediation or with therapeutic conversation, is not a matter of final mastery but of cultivating a sensitive awareness of how we are indeed multiply committed and drawn in different directions. We are always prone to getting stuck, to falling back into fixed beliefs about who we are, who are patients are, or what our role is.

Stories can get stuck, both for patients and for nurses. Labels are stories in bulk and they come at a discount. Labels are aberrant stories, with two dimensional characters and predictable endings, stories that are all spoilers. Labels are a falling back from emptiness into form, from the not-yet-determined into the known and secure. They are also part of a shared language – they would not work unless they were commonly understood. As such, they do more than reduce individuals to aggregate diagnoses seasoned with judgement, they are carriers of stories of mental health nursing. When we use labels we may be telling more about ourselves than about our patients.

Boundaries and borderlines

From a perspective of interconnectedness, boundaries are not simply an objective line that all can agree on and all can observe, or not. It may help to consider national boundaries, or frontiers as a metaphor for boundaries in the health care context. For one thing, this is a reminder that boundaries are only necessary where there is connection. Countries have to be adjacent to each other to share a frontier. They are both a marker of separation and of connection at the same time. The next observation is that there are frontiers and 'frontiers'. In the European Union, there is now very little control on the ground between many countries. That does not mean, however, that one cannot instantly tell when one has stepped from Germany into France, from one culture into another. At the opposite extreme, the frontier between North and South Korea is almost impermeable, with a separating demilitarized zone. Even here, at one of the world's politically harshest frontiers, there has been an unintended consequence that the no-man's land between the Korean states has become a de facto nature refuge for endangered species (Azios, 2008).

The frontier as metaphor demonstrates not only the ambivalence and variability of boundaries, but also that a boundary is both a real line and a symbolic judgement. Politically, judgement can be expressed in terms of the policies that make one frontier open (mostly) and another closed (mostly). Thus, returning to the nurse-patient relationship, although there are indeed real lines set out in our governing documents of practice, there are also judgements constantly being made and re-made about boundaries. The Canadian Nurses Association *Code of Ethics* (2017), for example, has a clear list of thou-shalt-nots.

> Nurses maintain appropriate professional boundaries and ensure their relationships are always for the benefit of the person. They recognize the potential vulnerability of persons receiving care and do not exploit their trust and dependency in a way that might compromise the therapeutic relationship. They do not abuse their relationship for personal or financial gain and do not enter into personal relationships (romantic, sexual or other) with persons receiving care.
>
> (see Honouring Dignity, point 7, p. 13)

By contrast, the *Standards of Practice* of the Canadian Federation of Mental Health Nurses (2014) include the element of judgement in the expectation that the nurse, who "Assesses and clarifies the influences of personal beliefs, values and life experience on the therapeutic relationship and distinguishes between social and therapeutic relationships" (p. 7).

Boundaries are important regulators of the interrelationships between nurses and patients, and a source of accountability for nurses as professionals. As with political borders, however, boundaries are a function of connection, and a negotiation between connection and separation. What to one person may be a clear boundary not to be crossed, to someone else can be a place of meeting and collaboration. If the latter point of view entails risk, and a lively judgement about what is appropriate and helpful, the former is no less a matter of judgement, but with less discernment and responsiveness. From the perspective of interconnectedness, boundaries become one of the conditioning elements of working therapeutically through relationship but are not an a priori determinant of practice.

"Make me one with everything": interconnection versus holism

Interconnection in the context of nursing practice might seem to lend itself to the idea that nursing is, or ought to be holistic. In one paper about holism in mental health, the characteristics of holism are explained as first, "identifying the interrelationships of the bio-psycho-social-spiritual dimensions of the person, recognizing that the whole is greater than the sum of its parts" and second, "understanding the individual as a unitary whole in mutual process with the environment" (Zahourek, 2008, p. 32). One of the difficulties of claims around holism is that there is no clear definition, although these are at least commonly held associations around the concept. Reed (2009), in a paper giving an overview of nursing theory at the turn of the twenty-first century, noted the prevalence of the term and complained, "Holism is a default term employed too often in place of clearer and more precise language to describe the perspective and unique contributions of nursing" (p. 103). One of the problems with the term when used to define nursing is that it seems perverse to deploy such apparently inclusive terminology to separate one's own discipline from all the others.

I propose, based on Buddhist thought, that the concept of interconnectedness is both more conceptually sound, and more helpful for establishing a basis for situated and flexible practice. First, it is true that there is a notion of oneness in Buddhism, alluded to in the joke about a Buddhist monk going up to a hot dog vendor and saying, "Make me one with everything!" The Buddhist idea of oneness, however, is not at the level of the whole person, or even the person interacting with the environment. Nishitani, a Japanese Buddhist philosopher, explained that there are two opposite and complementary ways of seeing the mind, from the self-centred view from which we each look out on the world, and from the "vantage point of 'the world'" (1982, p. 96). He wrote that, "the two ways of viewing the mind, cosmocentric and self-centric, have been inseparably preserved throughout Buddhism, in marked contrast to the West" (p. 96). What links and brings alive these ways of seeing is the idea of emptiness-as-plenitude, the radical interconnectedness that makes us part of the world and the world part of us.

The conventional definitions of holism, quoted above, fall short of such a philosophy of interconnection and retain assumptions of separation. The idea of the whole person, who is more than the sum of biological, psychological, social, and spiritual parts, for example is a building block metaphor of personhood. It is all very well to say more than the sum of parts, but if there is a claim to know the whole, then it must be possible to say exactly what the "more" consists of. Knowing the whole is also predicated on another, separate, knowing subject who can apprehend the whole person. This is a problematic claim. We never know ourselves entirely, let alone anyone else and there is something hubristic about even suggesting that we can.

The second part of the definition posits the person as "a unitary whole in mutual process with the environment" (Zahourek, 2008, p. 32). The argument against this in Buddhist thought is that if a person really is a unitary whole, then he or she cannot at the same time be in process with the environment, which implies conditionality and mutability (Garfield, 1995).

The great value of interconnectedness as opposed to holism is that it enjoins practice. We are inextricably and unavoidably bound up in the world, which we apprehend from the "self-centric" view as the changing situation of our lives, moment to moment. Using Buddhist terminology, a contemporary Western Zen teacher expressed it like this:

> Being willing to remain upright and still in the middle of the searing flames of life and of our garbled karma and conditioning, we can begin to settle into our deeper awareness which shows us the weave of our interconnections with all buddhas and sentient beings.
>
> (Leighton, 2003, p. 154)

Practicing as a nurse within the weave of interconnection is different from trying to know a whole person. It already acknowledges the impossibility of knowing the whole, and instead requires an active awareness of which connections matter in a given situation, and which connections can be helpfully addressed. To give an obvious example, a nurse meeting a patient who is bleeding internally in the emergency room will very quickly focus on certain actions, for example making the patient comfortable, monitoring blood pressure, and instigating steps towards urgent investigation and treatment. Another nurse at the same time might be concerned with contacting family, and the next day the priorities will have changed. This constant calibration of judgements about what needs to be done is the practice of interconnection. It does not preclude any of the supposed virtues of holism, that nurses may address numerous aspects of the patient's experience, or that it can lend a critical perspective to structures that predetermine or limit the scope of nurses' attention.

Finally, interconnection by definition cannot be claimed for one discipline. All that can be safely assumed is that different disciplines are likely to emphasize some lines of connection in a person's experience over others. This standpoint is more congenial to being able to appreciate difference while finding ground for collaboration than hoisting the banner of holism over nursing.

This, however, is where the philosophical rigour of the Buddhist tradition is important. Although interconnection is posited as a condition of being, with the concomitant effects that things (including concepts and our sense of self) are impermanent and always changing there is also the fundamental recognition of our everyday assumptions of wanting some things to stay the same and others to go away. It is in this tension between the two views that practice arises, in the endless effort to apprehend the present moment and to act for the benefit of self and others. This basic structure of practice within the midst of things, which encompasses the difficulty of human life and yet upholds compassion as an ethical imperative has great potential value to how nurses think about nursing.

Conclusion

What has caught the attention of Westerners in Buddhist thought is its seeming relevance to our modern condition, to "liquid modernity" in the phrase of the sociologist Zygmunt Bauman (2000). It has elements of existential concern with the immediate presences of daily living, an orientation towards suffering as part of the human condition, combined with an ethical call to compassion. If all of these elements are partly what we most want to find in Buddhism, that does not mean that they are not legitimately parts of the tradition, nor that there is anything wrong with the inflection of Asian traditions with Western movements of thought. One of the strengths of the humanities in general, which includes religious thought, is that invite different ways of relating to time and progress, and speak to us in the here and now across centuries. Part of the fascination of works of ancient art and literature is that those that have survived have often done so because they continue to resonate. I will conclude with a Zen koan, which happens to mention nursing in this English translation. It is beyond the scope of this chapter to attempt to understand the function of these brief, enigmatic exchanges in Zen monastic training. But for a modern, secular, nursing reader, there is something here about unsettling fixed definitions of sickness and health, of the health of the health care provider, and of the urgency to do something anyway, because the world will not wait for the answer ...

> Attention! Isan asked Dogo, "Where have you been?" Dogo said, "I've been nursing." Isan said, "How many people were sick?" Dogo replied, "Some are sick, some are not." Isan pursued, "Isn't it you who's not sick?" Dogo responded, "Sickness and nonsickness have nothing at all to do with *it*. Speak quickly! Speak quickly!" Isan remarked, "Even being able to say it misses entirely."
>
> (Wick, 2005, p. 262)

Note

1 McMahan uses the term "Buddhist modernism" because he points out that Buddhist adaptation to modernity has also happened in traditionally Buddhist societies. I have stuck with the terminology of Western Buddhism, since it reflects my contact with Buddhist ideas and practices refracted largely through Western teachers and writers.

References

Azios, T. (2008, 21 November). Korean demilitarized zone now a wildlife haven. *Christian Science Monitor*. Retrieved from www.csmonitor.com

Barker, P., & Buchanan-Barker, P. (2005). *The Tidal Model: A guide for mental health professionals*. New York, NY: Brunner-Routledge.

Bauman, Z. (2000). *Liquid modernity*. London, UK: Wiley.

Bruce, A. (2007). (Time)lessness: Buddhist perspectives and end-of-life. *Nursing Philosophy, 8*, 151–157. doi: 10.1111/j.1466-769X.2007.00310.x

Buswell, R.E., & Lopez, D.S. (2014). *The Princeton dictionary of Buddhism.* Princeton, NJ: Princeton University Press.

Canadian Federation of Mental Health Nurses. (2014). *Canadian standards for psychiatric-mental health nursing: Standards of practice* (4th ed.). Toronto, ON, Canada: Author.

Canadian Nurses Association. (2017). *Code of ethics for registered nurses.* Retrieved from www.cna-aiic.ca/en/nursing-practice/nursing-ethics#toc

Garfield, J. (1995). *The fundamental wisdom of the middle way: Nagarjuna's mulamadhyamakakarika.* New York, NY: Oxford University Press.

Joy, M. (2011). *After appropriation: Explorations in intercultural philosophy and religion.* Calgary, AB, Canada: University of Calgary.

Kabat-Zinn, J. (1990). *Full catastrophe living: Using the wisdom of your body and mind to face stress, pain, and illness.* New York, NY: Delta.

Leighton, T.D. (2003). *Faces of compassion: Classic bodhisattva archetypes and their modern expression.* Boston, MA: Wisdom.

Lopez, D.S. (Ed.). (2004). *Buddhist scriptures.* London, UK: Penguin.

McCaffrey, G., Raffin-Bouchal, S., & Moules, N.J. (2012). Buddhist thought and nursing: A hermeneutic exploration. *Nursing Philosophy, 13,* 87–97.

McMahan, D.L. (2008). *The making of Buddhist modernism.* New York, NY: Oxford University Press.

Nhat Hanh, T. (2006). *Understanding our mind.* Berkeley, CA: Parallax.

Nhat Hanh, T. (2008). *Peaceful action, open heart: Lessons from the Lotus Sutra.* Berkeley, CA: Parallax.

Nishijima, G., & Cross, C. (2006). *Master Dogen's Shobogenzo: Book 1.* www.dogen sangha.org

Nishitani, K. (1982). *Religion and nothingness* (J. van Bragt trans.). Berkeley, CA: University of California Press.

Poirier, M.R. (2016). Mischief in the marketplace for mindfulness. In R. Rosenbaum & B. Magid (Eds.), *What's wrong with mindfulness (and what isn't): Zen perspectives* (pp. 13–28). Somerville, MA: Wisdom.

Reed, P.G. (2009). Nursing reformation: Historical reflections and philosophic foundations. In P. Reed & N. Crawford-Shearer (Eds.), *Perspectives on nursing theory* (pp. 100–107). Philadelphia, PA: Wolters Kluwer/Lippincott Williams & Wilkins.

Rich, K. (2007). Using a Buddhist sangha as a model of communitarianism in nursing. *Nursing Ethics, 14,* 466–477. doi: 10.1177/0969733007077881

Rich, K. (2010). No essence no self: Using a Buddhist perspective to characterize the nature of nursing. *Advances in Nursing Science, 33*(4), 344–351.

Rizzetto, D.E. (2005). *Waking up to what you do.* Boston, MA: Shambhala.

Rodgers, B., & Yen, W.-J. (2002). Re-thinking nursing science through the understanding of Buddhism. *Nursing Philosophy, 3,* 213–221. doi: 10.1046/j.1466-769X.2002.00105.x

Smith H., & Novak, P. (2004). *Buddhism: A concise introduction.* New York, NY: HarperCollins.

Wick, G.S. (2005). *The book of equanimity: Illuminating classic Zen koans.* Boston, MA: Wisdom.

Zahourek, R.P. (2008). Integrative holism in psychiatric-mental health nursing. *Journal of Psychosocial Nursing, 46*(10), 31–37.

9 Nursing and humanities in the age of the post-human

In this chapter, I look at the future of the relationship between nursing and the humanities. Just as the humanities have adapted over the centuries in response to changes in economic and social conditions, so will their relationship with nursing, which will continue to be modulated by what is happening to the profession as part of health care more broadly. First, I will consider these broader trends, then focus in the role of the humanities. My overarching image is the cyborg (Clark, 2003; Haraway, 1985/2016), the combination of human and machine. Far from making the humanities redundant, multiple possibilities in the cyborg future (and present) create a vital space for the imaginative, creative, and impassioned mapping of the shifting borders of the human.

Nursing and technology

As we saw at the start of this book, the formation of modern nursing runs alongside modern scientific medicine and its breakthrough technologies of anaesthesia and antisepsis. Nursing has, out of necessity, developed in lockstep with technological changes so that, with variations by specialty, the work of nursing is infused with technical knowledge and skills, and is mediated by sophisticated machines. If there is a shift in the boundary between human and technological that is central to nursing, it is this: technology has already moved beyond the model of tools manipulated by humans and into the human body itself. Medical technology is still about machines that do things to people, but increasingly it is becoming about intimate integrations of technology and manipulation of the human substance itself. Heart pacemakers have been around as an accessible intervention for about 50 years. By modern standards it is a fairly crude device to augment natural human functioning, but it is an important marker of the shifting boundary between human and artificial, in the form of a piece of equipment that safely resides within the body. Current advances in medical science are happening in areas of robotics, nanotechnology, artificial intelligence, and genetics, all of which push at the boundary between human and technological. Genetics is a case of technology being brought to bear on the basic matter of human development and identity. If high-tech external aids might alter a person's sense of self-in-the-world, technological manipulation of genes can affect the original formation of a sense of self.

(Another border coming into sight in medical science that is not between machine and human is that between body tissue and microbiome. Research into the human microbiome, the microbacterial environment that pervades the human body, disrupts the boundary between self and non-self at the biological level. "I is another" in the French poet Rimbaud's (1871/2002, p. 572) famous phrase turns out to be a biological observation.)

Nursing, as it has since the nineteenth century, has to contend with technological change but now, as for human beings in general, with changes that have profound implications for the limits of the human itself. The significance of these trends for nursing is where they work along the borderlines between the human and the technological, in the territory of the cyborg.

The cyborg concept

A cyborg is an organism combining machine and biological entities. Familiar from science fiction, in films like *RoboCop*, the term dates back to 1960, short for "cybernetic organism" (O'Connell, 2017, p. 142). It was coined by a neurophysiologist and a physician who wrote a paper speculating that the human organism would have to be adapted by technology to travel in space. An underlying assumption of cybernetics, written into the concept of the cyborg, is that humans and other animals are information processing beings, so that the metaphor of machine logic is inscribed into the human from the outset (O'Connell, 2017). Donna Haraway introduced the idea of the cyborg in the context of feminist and socialist critique in 1985 in her much-quoted *Cyborg Manifesto* (2016). Although dated in some respects, she opened up the idea of the cyborg beyond the narrow limits of specific technical applications to explore its potential ramifications in socio-cultural life. Early on she noted the spillage of terms like information and coding from the realms of computing to biology and society. Humans are genetically coded, concatenations of information: "organisms have ceased to exist as objects of knowledge, giving way to biotic components, i.e., Special kinds of information-processing devices" (p. 35). This, from 1985, is prescient. The image of the cyborg stands for more than examples of human-technical interface such as a pacemaker or a smartphone; it is a far-reaching metaphor for changes to how humans encounter themselves and the world. One example, rapidly becoming familiar to nursing students, is the use of simulation in practice education, reaching out to touch future patients through sophisticated veils of simulacra. New borders, of flesh and machine, of virtual and actual have become part of everyday experience. In cyborgs, "there is an intimate experience of boundaries, their construction and deconstruction" (Haraway, 2016, p. 66). Her point about boundaries thrown into question is crucial for nursing and the humanities.

More recently, Andy Clark (2003), a philosopher of embodied cognition, has argued that humans have always been cyborgs, in the sense that tools have always been a mode of external extension of human capacities. The borderline between the human and the technological has existed since a proto-human manipulated an object as a tool for the first time. Yuval Noah Harari (2016) in a high-level survey of the history of humankind as a species, traces the presence of technology in societal imaginaries and its effects on human lives and environments. Since the Industrial Revolution, the power of technology has accelerated exponentially such that geologists now debate naming a new planetary epoch, the Anthropocene, for the ineradicable marks left on the Earth by human activity (Davison, 2019). While some geologists resist the idea of marking a new era within living memory, advocates of the Anthropocene argue over exactly when it began. One candidate is 1945 with the first human-made atomic explosions that have left a layer of radioactive fallout in the Earth's surface.

Nonetheless, one of the signs of the Anthropocene is that the borderline between human and tool now moves exponentially more quickly than in any previous era. Human-tool interaction or cyborg life, as Clark (2003) argues, is a cultural as well as a bio-technical phenomenon. Cyborg ways of life are emerging, based upon rapid movements of immense amounts of data and characterized by constant arrays of images, with staccato bursts of language, abbreviated and punctuated with symbols. Theorists of nursing have long argued that nurses ought to be environmentally attuned to care for patients in the full conditions of their lives as it relates to some or other presenting health problem. That attunement now includes the techno-socio-political landscapes of contemporary life.

Borderlines of the cyborg age pass through healthcare literally, in the form of bodies augmented by technical devices, and in Clark's extended sense in the uses of technologies of monitoring, life support, information processing, remote communication, and virtual imaging. Every area of nursing is affected, leading to discussion of how to characterize and how best to manage work at the borders of the human and the technological (Archibald & Barnard, 2017; Barnard & Sandelowski, 2001; Lapum et al., 2012; Monteiro, 2016; Sandelowski, 2002). Lapum et al. (2012) take the step of naming a "cyborg ontology" (p. 279) to begin to come to terms with the extent and pace of technological presence in nursing life, and to define "the liminal space between technology and [person centred care]" (p. 279). They find a potential balance between the human and technological sides of cyborg nursing, which requires the proper precision and repeatability of much care (knowing the important of timing and dosage in giving medications, for example), along with a capacity to move into relational spaces of un-programmable possibility between people. They note how social environments are organized to reflect the model of technological regularity and how many nurses' "actions and behaviours are mediated by technology" (p. 282). Archibald and Barnard prefer the term "posthumanism" (p. 2476) to capture the way that technology permeates our lives, our environments, our ways of thinking to a profound extent. They too want to get away from a position of opposing technology to humane caring through "coalescence", recognizing that "technology is inseparable from care and humanity" (p. 2474). They argue that nurses ought to be looking deliberatively to the future to work out how best to work with technology. Sandelowski (2002) relates borderlines to themes already present in nursing about distinctions between "body work and information work" (p. 67) where there is a traditional ambivalence towards the former, seen as low status, dirty work, while the latter has been valued as more sophisticated and more professional. Even the language of "the interpersonal" (p. 62) puts nursing into the space between bodies. Hence new technical affordances such as telehealth may reproduce a tendency towards disembodiment and invisibility of nursing work, which is also, as she points out regarded as women's work. Sandelowski frames desired reconciliation in cyborg nursing as seeing "body and information work as constituting each other, and the body as a source of knowledge and power for nursing" (p. 68).

Science and technology determine the forward frontiers of cyborg existence, while the social sciences rush to keep up with the pace of change. But science comes from an already existing mesh of assumptions, values, and affordances, not to mention imaginative projections, that tend to become hidden in the flash and glitter of each novel finding or technical innovation. The humanities are the field of the imagination in which we read ourselves back to ourselves, work out how we got to where we are, and formulate ideas of where we might be headed. In the following sections, I consider examples of rapidly moving borderlines that affect nursing's imaginaries: robotics, health surveillance, and futurist projections about life and death themselves in the movement known as Transhumanism. Within these trends, however, the stubborn human element demands expression.

Nurse-robots

Robots are machines designed and built to carry out programmed tasks. They are already making inroads into traditional nursing tasks, the borderline of "human-robot interaction" (Metzler & Barnes, 2014, p. 4) is already moving fast. Archibald and Barnard (2017) list examples of robots that specialize in feeding people, robotic bathtubs that automatically soap and shower their occupants, robots that can transfer patients into bed, and robots that provide companionship and advice. It is not projecting too far into the future to imagine a combination robot that can take on all those roles, plus monitoring vital signs and administering medication. It is simple to find videos online of robots in nursing homes (see for example Hamstra, 2018) serving as companions to residents, providing easy video communication with family members, or a tactile, comforting presence. It is no surprise that many of these innovations are coming from Japan, which has a robust electronics sector and an ageing population without the mitigation of large scale immigration to maintain the labour pool. In short, Japanese society needs carers without having a large group of workers willing to take low paid, low status positions. Questions about how much should robots be doing for residents in nursing homes are as likely to be answered by technological capacity and economies of scale as ethical notions of what good care means.

Along the borderline of the real and the synthetic, smiling robots might reliably offer physical assistance while also creating a sense of comfort and safety in the patient. And if it *feels* like being cared for to those on the receiving end, is that not caring? (Metzler & Barnes, 2014). Just as people have quickly become accustomed to communication taking place via messaging perhaps we will take readily to automated care environments. The human touch is held up as one of the distinctive traits of nursing that makes it invulnerable to machine replacement. However, in the cyborg age, even human touch is moving along with borders between humans and machines. For nurses, this should be a call to sharpen ethical thinking, to be realistic about the kinds of choices that are already upon us in health care, to anticipate those that are coming, and to advocate for nurses to go on providing what is uniquely human in concert with technology.

Data, surveillance, self-surveillance

Monitoring, surveillance, and data collection have always been central to nurses' work (Sandelowski, 2000). At the individual level, nurses make systematic observations of patients starting with the basics of temperature, pulse, and respiration rate, and record their findings. Within a generation, the process has gone from skin-to-skin contact, direct observation, and basic technology of mercury thermometers[1] to electronic measurement; from recording findings using pen and paper filed in a chart, to electronic storage and accompanying ease of data distribution throughout health information networks. At the community level, surveillance is part of public health nursing practice, collecting, interpreting and reporting on health-related data (World Health Organization, 2019). Surveillance in health care, tracking disease outbreaks, identifying high risk individuals, predicting population health trends, and crafting individual treatment plans is increasingly driven by big data. Immense amounts of health data are now generated constantly and it is only a matter of developing usable analytic tools to keep up. Data comes from sources within health care systems, from electronic health records, medication prescribing, diagnostic imaging and as well from dispersed machines living alongside patients, social media, and health apps (Raghupathi & Raghupathi, 2014).

One aspect of big data that is new, beyond the sheer scale and movability of data, is input from personal devices. Self-surveillance is a technological phenomenon, an affordance for health care practitioners, a socio-political issue, and an existential question. Next generation cyborgs are beings not only of biological and non-biological materials but of distributed data, self-referential, and self-surveillant. Data is generated by oneself and available to oneself, but via unseen networks furnished by corporate entities (I was surprised recently to find a friend of mine on another continent sending me "kudos" for my bike rides recorded on the Strava app). Self-surveillance technology renders us differently to ourselves, presenting our bodies back as data about steps taken, heart and respiration rates, or blood sugar level. As controversies surrounding Facebook have revealed, surface claims of tech corporations may conceal the acquisition and buying and selling of data. Whose data, and for what purposes? Insurance companies have started to offer incentives to customers willing to hand over data from personal fitness devices (Ingraham, 2018). While health care organizations work with established ideas of confidentiality and privacy, it is increasingly difficult to control flows of data among individuals, health care institutions, insurance companies, and social media where it is not even clear any longer what constitutes health information.

Sandelowski refers to modern clinical practice, that uses communications and imaging technology to span outer and inner space, as "an array of spectacular encounters" (2002, p. 66). It is an intriguing choice of words that has echoes of Guy Debord, the instigator of the art-political movement of Situationism, who published his best-known work, the *Society of the Spectacle* in 1967. In it, he proposed that advanced capitalism created an all embracing "spectacle through which social relationships are mediated" (Gray, 2016). Not only has Debord's Society of the Spectacle flourished beyond his imagining, but we have ingested it whole, we are become a spectacle unto ourselves. As Gray notes, "If the technology through which surveillance operates also provides continuous entertainment, [people] may soon find any other way of living intolerable" (p. 125). Wearable fitness devices and the data they generate are a new hybrid spectacle of health, entertainment, self-expression, and potential for manipulation and control.

Even mindfulness, that ancient and most un-technological of practices (noticing your own breath is about all that is required), is framed as a technique of self-monitoring, scanning for negative thoughts that might impede one's self-esteem or productivity. Through classes, apps, and workplace health schemes, mindfulness has become a global industry, built literally on air (Poirier, 2016). Whereas some critics are inclined to blame the messenger and condemn mindfulness as a neoliberal trick to render people into willing circuits in corporate machines (Purser, 2019), mindfulness is only a mirror for social trends, just as for centuries it was a mirror to the Buddhist aspiration to nirvana in Asian societies. Mindfulness can just as well make for more clear-thinking anti-capitalist activists as for more alert lawyers, nurses, or drone operators. Mindfulness is morally neutral. It is a method for altering consciousness, with effects of reducing random noise in the mind and clarifying attention, but it has nothing to say about which objects of attention to choose. In contact with Western preoccupations, however, it has become harnessed to a self-involved, aspirational desire for wellness that is the opposite of its traditional association with quieting the appetites of the ego.

Health monitoring and surveillance have become all-pervasive and ever-present, in a world where personal fitness devices, intimately tracking feet and hearts, are linked through mediating layers to vast swarms of data. Unseen in those layers are the structures, motivations, needs, and desires of clinicians, researchers, governments, and corporations. By means of the humanities, whether through research or creative endeavour, we can track ourselves tracking ourselves, tracing unnoticed networks of influence.

Transhumanism

At the further reaches of human transformation are advocates for transhumanism, an umbrella term for those who enthusiastically look for ways of transcending human being as we know it (O'Connell, 2017). In his entertaining book about his travels among the transhumanists, Mark O'Connell recounts meetings with a variety of people seeking to transcend the limits of human life as we have known it up to now. They include entrepreneurs in Silicon Valley who offer cryogenic freezing of brains against the day one's self can be uploaded into another kind of vessel (there is a full body version available for those who might doubt the brain-in-jar hypothesis); scientists who have declared ageing unnatural and death an outrage, who believe in the indefinite extension of the lifespan; and believers in the coming Singularity, when artificial intelligence will overleap its human creators and morph into as yet unknowable forms of hyper-intelligent techno-life. Transhumanism seems remote from nursing concerns but it is worth considering for two reasons. First, it already appears in bioethics literature as exerting pressure on ethics through questioning the hitherto accepted limits of the human (Lawrence, 2017; Porter, 2017). This is another point on the cyborg frontier. Bio, meaning life and biology, is the study of living things, resting on a deep assumption that there is an unassimilable divide between living and inanimate things. Mergings of flesh and machine envisaged in transhumanist futures throw into question the divide itself. Second, although transhumanism is, at least for now, a fringe movement it shows in extreme form trends that are already filtering into the mainstream. It is not news from nowhere and if it is not a reliable guide to the future, it may be some kind of guide to the present.

Transhumanism is at one extreme of the advocacy of technological progress. For transhumanists, progress is not only inevitable and desirable, but the fulfilment of human reason. In this, it is like a turbo-charged version of Enlightenment thinking, stripped of nuance. Transhumanist thinking often has a blind spot of not being able to see its own moral biases, taking them to be universally shared human values. Transhumanists all seem to envisage an oddly frictionless future in which human conflicts of values and goals somehow disappear. There is an ominous gap between our present and the post-human future, leaving out the economic and political mechanisms by which we are supposed to get there. Some transhumanist writing sounds libertarian, lionizing individual achievement if only the state would get out of the way, but naively ignoring the role of private corporations. There is also something solipsistic about transhumanist thinking. Whose brain is worth freezing? Who should live forever? If the answer is an egalitarian everybody, it raises obvious quibbles about overcrowding once the most natural population control of death is removed, never mind more philosophical concerns about the value of life arising from its finitude. However, it seems more likely it is the advocates of transhumanist solutions themselves who picture their own existence as most essential to humanity in perpetuity. General de Gaulle once remarked, "the graveyards are full of indispensable men" – perhaps too, the backs of fridges in Silicon Valley.

Transhumanism is a curious amalgam of an exorbitant anthropocentrism for which the universe finds its ultimate meaning in human data extraction, with a cheerful longing for an end to humanity itself, since the human in the end is only a means to the data extraction, good enough while it lasts, like last year's iPhone, until a new version comes along. Nursing on this reading is doomed to disappear but since it will do so along with the human race as we currently know it, that hardly seems important. However, we do not need to achieve anything like a post-human state to detect a shift in human attitudes towards health and death, born partly from the wild successes of medical science to date, and partly from the formation of the citizen-consumer who expects technical assistance to fix the device, even if that device happens to be a bodily organ. There is a new Cartesianism in the air, where body and mind are resolutely separate and the body can be worked upon, adjusted, added to or subtracted from, at the behest of the controlling mind (and with the goodwill and hands of willing surgeons of course). Our new situation gives rise to unexpected alliances, where the most emphatic religious believers may also be the most willing to accept completely non-natural interventions to keep alive bodies from which most brain activity has irrevocably departed.

Nurses need to keep their heads about them, need to read across variant interpretations of the human, to hold on to the possible – what is scientifically possible, what is at any given moment politically, economically, and ethically possible, what it is possible to imagine and what it is possible to believe, even in spite of the evidence. The play of possibility around the embodied human person that has always been and, for now at least, remains the central focus of nursing work needs the humanities every bit as much as science.

Back to nursing and humanities

A British philosopher John Gray remarked, "… if you want a glimpse of what a post-human future would be like, read Homer" (2016). For the foreseeable future, not only will human beings continue to strive and suffer while pursuing innumerable different ways of living, so there will continue to be a need for nursing to make its contribution to health and the alleviation of suffering. Gray's comment points to the way in which great works of literature or art continue to speak to us, and continue to convey messages that are profound and immediate, even across great cultural and historical distances. Some things do not change, and we are destined to go on rediscovering them anew. This is the Archimedean point of leverage of the humanities. The future for humanities and nursing is in securing the importance of embodied, enculturated, human experience when matters of health are at stake. Humanities give ways to make sense of human experience through stories and images, through research and teaching that make use of stories and images. Nursing intersects with the human along points where questions of health are at stake, where new borders have appeared on the map, and borders are constantly shifting. Nurses work on borderlines of the human, inside the cyborg world. But the cyborg future is still a human future, of communication and miscommunication, of root networks of desires and fears, of felt embodied experience, of symbolism and metaphor. Nursing without the humanities is not nursing at all. It is robotics.

Technology, education, and nursing

Technology has such immense power and prestige that it exerts a gravitational pull on how people see and think about the world, beyond its immediate applications. This is true of education as much as anywhere else, where STEM disciplines (Science, Technology, Engineering, and Mathematics) now enjoy hegemony. Of course, as I have argued, modern nursing requires something from all these areas and yet is not reducible to any of them. Practice disciplines in general, such as social work and education as well as nursing, do not indeed fit easily into the traditional bipolar academy of humanities and sciences. (Medicine and law, by dint of long-established prestige, are accepted as occupying their own unquestioned space.)

Rather than having to seek identity in one (almost always science) or the other it makes more sense to value and explore what it is to be in an intermediary, mixed space, where practice precedes prejudices belonging to traditional forms of education. And yet, of course, nursing as a discipline of higher education is subject to wider trends shaping universities. Demand for STEM is combined with political and economic forces. In a recent paper, writing from his experience of the UK university system, Rolfe (2019) tracks the history of the university as an institution, noting that nursing entered the academy just as it turned towards its current business-model incarnation where the market and the creation of student-as-consumer have overtaken autonomous academic values. The result of this for nursing is that academics are torn between conflicting demands, "between giving the customers what they *want* in order for them to secure well-paid employment, and giving them what they *need* in order to be caring, compassionate and effective nurses" (Rolfe, 2019, p. 7). His suggested solution is a strategy of "subversion", to find ways of balancing both sets of demands within the world of the corporate university, and that to do so is to behave philosophically, to think actively about where we find ourselves, what is demanded of us, what we desire, and how to live.

I extend Rolfe's proposal from philosophy to the humanities more generally. It is not only a question of thinking but of seeing, feeling, and experiencing, of responding to the multitudinous ways in which life makes demands of human beings. The work of the humanities has always endeavoured to respond in kind, through art, poetry, history, and storytelling as well as philosophical thinking. So far, so eternal – there is no sign yet of the human need for meaning and value, and contestations of meaning and value, going away.

Note

1 Random nostalgic note: younger nurses will never know the experience of chasing tiny balls of mercury from a broken thermometer around the floor.

References

Archibald, M.M., & Barnard, A. (2017). Futurism in nursing: Technology, robotics, and the fundamentals of care. *Journal of Clinical Nursing*, *27*, 2473–2480. doi: 10.1111/jocn.14081.

Barnard, A., & Sandelowski, M. (2001). Technology and humane nursing care: (Ir)reconcilable or invented difference? *Journal of Advanced Nursing, 34*(3), 367–375.

Clark, A. (2003). *Natural-born cyborgs: Minds, technologies, and the future of human intelligence.* Oxford, UK: Oxford University Press.

Davison, N. (2019). The Anthropocene epoch: Have we entered a new phase of planetary history? *The Guardian,* 30 May 2019. Retrieved from www.theguardian.com/environment/2019/may/30/anthropocene-epoch-have-we-entered-a-new-phase-of-planetary-history

Gray, J. (2016). Humanity mk II: Why the future of humanity will be just as purposeless as the past. *New Statesman,* 22 September 2016. Retrieved from www.newstatesman.com/culture/books/2016/10/humanity-mk-ii-why-future-humanity-will-be-just-purposeless-past

Hamstra, B. (2018). Will these nurse robots take your job? Don't freak out just yet. *nurse. org.* Retrieved from https://nurse.org/articles/nurse-robots-friend-or-foe/

Haraway, D. (2016). *Manifestly Haraway.* Minneapolis, MN: University of Minnesota Press.

Ingraham, C. (2018). An insurance company wants you to hand over your Fitbit data so it can make more money. Should you? *Washington Post,* 25 September 2018. Retrieved from www.washingtonpost.com/business/2018/09/25/an-insurance-company-wants-you-hand-over-your-fitbit-data-so-they-can-make-more-money-should-you/?noredirect=on&utm_term=.9228c0f39770

Lapum, J., Fredericks, S., Beanlands, H., McCay, E., Schwind, J., & Romaniuk, D. (2012). A cyborg ontology in health care: Traversing into the liminal space between technology and person-centred practice. *Nursing Philosophy, 13,* 276–288.

Lawrence, D.R. (2017). The edge of human? The problem with the posthuman as the "beyond". *Bioethics, 31*(3), 171–179. doi: 10.1111/bioe.12318

Metzler, T.A., & Barnes, S.J. (2014). Three dialogues concerning robots in elder care. *Nursing Philosophy, 15,* 4–13. doi: 10.1111/nup.12027

Monteiro, A.P.T.A.V.M. (2016). Cyborgs, biotechnologies, and informatics in health care – New paradigms in nursing sciences. *Nursing Philosophy, 17,* 19–27. doi: 10.1111/nup.12088

O'Connell, M. (2017). *To be a machine: Adventures among cyborgs, utopians, hackers, and the futurists solving the modest problem of death.* London, UK: Granta.

Poirier, M.R. (2016). Mischief in the marketplace for mindfulness. In R. Rosenbaum & B. Magid (Eds.), *What's wrong with mindfulness (and what isn't): Zen perspectives* (pp. 13–28). Somerville, MA: Wisdom.

Porter, A. (2017). Bioethics and transhumanism. *Journal of Medicine and Philosophy, 42,* 237–260. doi: 10.1093/jmp/jhx001

Purser, R. (2019). The mindfulness conspiracy. *The Guardian,* 14 June 2019. Retrieved from www.theguardian.com/lifeandstyle/2019/jun/14/the-mindfulness-conspiracy-capitalist-spirituality

Raghupathi, W., & Raghupathi, V. (2014). Big data analytics in healthcare: Promise and potential. *Health Information Science and Systems, 2*(3), 1–10.

Rimbaud, A. (2002). *Rimbaud complete* (W. Mason Ed. & Trans.). New York, NY: Modern Library.

Rolfe, G. (2019). Carry on thinking: Nurse education in the corporate university. *Nursing Philosophy,* 2019;00:e12270. doi: 10.1111/nup.12270

Sandelowski, M. (2000). *Devices & desires: Gender, technology, and American nursing.* Chapel Hill, NC: University of North Carolina Press.

Sandelowski, M. (2002). Visible humans, vanishing bodies, and virtual nursing: Complications of life, presence, place, and identity. *Advances in Nursing Science, 24*(3), 58–70.

World Health Organization. (2019). *Public health surveillance*. Retrieved from www.who.int/topics/public_health_surveillance/en/

Conclusion

In writing about nursing and the humanities, I have been trying to answer questions about why humanities belong in the ecology of nursing knowledge, and where they fit. Ecology is a fashionable metaphor but it seems like the right one to use for a hybrid profession like nursing, whose character lies precisely in its diversity, its borrowings and adaptations from other disciplines, and its constantly renewed work in caring for the health needs of others. I have traced the history of humanities and nursing, which is at the same time abundant but often defined differently than in the explicitly named field of medical humanities. Humanities have found a home in educational practices, nursing theory and philosophy, and in at least some forms of qualitative research without coalescing into a unified field, and usually unnoticed as humanities. Our attention, as a discipline, has often been directed into concerns about caring, or what we mean by art and evidence. Humanities have never quite fitted with the moral and spiritual demands of some commentators, nor with those who are sceptical of anything outside of pure scientific evidence. I hope we are getting better at taking an ecological view, recognizing the ways in which multiple kinds of knowledge need to flourish for nurses to find the full extent of their hybrid practices. That entails being good at telling apart worthwhile knowledge from worthless, or even dangerous knowledge. That in turn requires knowing criteria of rigour in different realms, and knowing which to apply where. That is why I have paid attention to the importance of science for nursing in a book about the humanities. It is all very well to talk about ecology of knowledge, and to celebrate hybridity, but there is a special responsibility in practice disciplines, which are centrally oriented towards obligation to those we serve, for carefully parsing what we know and how we practice.

In choosing certain themes, and emphasizing certain ways of explaining how humanities fit with nursing, I have traced only one path through the topic. There are many other ways to address the relationship between humanities and nursing. Over the course of writing the book, I have become aware of how, inevitably, my pathway reflects my own formation during a 35-year career in nursing and my education even before entering nursing.

I have written about areas I have studied, and that I am drawn to. I took a degree in history before becoming a nurse, and it seemed natural that I should write about the historical roots of nursing and the humanities. More than that, I have realized how much an early training in history has informed my work as a nurse over the years: gathering facts, evaluating sources, constructing accounts that make sense of the facts – while holding on the knowledge that you may not have all the facts, but you have to make your best judgement about what to do next.

I knew early on in my nurse education that I wanted to work in mental health. It is not the only reason, but I was very impressed that the first thing our instructor for our mental health module had us do was sit down and watch *One Flew Over the Cuckoo's Nest*. That was a good way to start thinking about mental health, nurses, and institutions. Mental health appealed to me as a specialty – and still does – because it relies on interpretation, of words and behaviours, of the changing descriptors of disorders in the DSM, of values and meanings, and even basic sensory perceptions. I went to work at the Cassel Hospital in the UK, a therapeutic community that had evolved out of the great innovations in group psychotherapy following World War II. It was an intense place to work – nurses engaged with patients constantly around practical tasks of running the community of around 50 people, and dealing with problems of relating that ensued. We used words, words, and more words – rooted in psychodynamic traditions, the life of the community fed into elaborate structures of sessions conducted by psychotherapists, with layers of community meetings run by patients and nurses, constantly striving to make sense of the moving life of the community. I learned the therapeutic power of language at the Cassel, making and unmaking meanings with patients, striving to help them find better ways of relating and coping.

Later on, when I started my graduate education in Canada in 2007, I was introduced to hermeneutic research for the first time by Dr. Nancy Moules, a leading scholar in the field. With its stress on history, language, dialogue, and interpretation hermeneutics was a good fit with the ways I had always thought about nursing and especially my field of mental health nursing. I have since used hermeneutics as a research approach, written about it and taught it. I was first introduced to the idea of carnal hermeneutics in 2011, when the philosopher Richard Kearney was the visiting scholar at the Canadian Hermeneutic Institute. Renewed attention to embodiment in hermeneutics has been my gateway to thinking anew about bodies in nursing, how they affect each other, the spaces in which they move, and the ways we can try to escape or ignore them.

Not long after completing my final chapter, I attended a nursing philosophy conference in Victoria, Canada where I heard presentations from nurses, and some philosophers, who are passionate about the power of ideas to influence how nursing develops into the future. (In the context of this book, it is worth pointing out that a nursing philosophy conference already embraces the humanities in nursing.) Among the great range of topics under discussion, I noticed a number that included the word materiality. At that meeting of people looking hard at what is going on in nursing, there did appear to be something in the air about reasserting the centrality of embodiment, of actual people in actual physical surroundings, in a call-and-response of nursing care for patients. This, of course, alongside another theme of what we are to make of artificial intelligence, wearable technologies, and big data (Risling, 2017). The old antinomy of flesh and spirit has a modern analogue in the material and the virtual. Interaction between the two is alive and well in contemporary nurses' thinking. There is something urgently new about the terms of the interaction, as technology changes rapidly, and something ancient about humans with our physical affordances and limitations manoeuvring inside powerful imaginaries that influence our lives.

Throughout my nursing career, I have turned to literature, poetry, and art as places where I can find solidarity in moments of strong emotion, sometimes clarity and sometimes shared puzzlement, beauty, consolation, and inspiration. To me, they are a part of my navigation through life, including my work as a nurse and now as a teacher and researcher of nursing. I realize that is not the case for everyone but it is not only a matter of personal taste either. The arts and humanities have always been how human societies have affirmed and reflected upon what matters to them; from handprints outlined in red chalk on cave walls 30,000 years ago, to the power plays of *Game of Thrones*. This is one of the roots of the importance of humanities for nursing.

In accounting for what I have covered in this book, I am aware too of things I have not addressed. I have written about poetry and prose but only mentioned other modes of artistic representation, such as music, painting, sculpture, drama, or film. There is, of course, endless scope to explore nodes of connection between artistic works and nursing. It would be wonderful to see another book (or multimedia website) that brought together examples of all kinds of artistic works, by and about and for nurses and those they care for.

Another area I have not emphasized is the critical potentiality of the humanities. This has been taken up well in recent works in medical and health humanities. Bleakley (2015) sees "democratizing medical culture" (p. 58) as the chief purpose for medical humanities, by exposing power differentials and upsetting assumptions about how things are, and how they could be. He warns against the palliative, or soothing, side of humanities that can fall into the trap of prettifying things that should not be prettified. One only needs to think of the socio-political context of widening wealth inequality, climate change, and pressures to reduce public health care provision, to see he has a point. Jones, Wear, and Friedman (2014) take a similar stance in their collection about the health humanities, which includes sections organized by, "gender and sexuality", "race and class", and "patient–professional relationships". (pp. vi–vii). Social justice and sensitivity to power structures are parts of the ecology of nursing knowledge that give nurses a lot to offer to critically-oriented health humanities. I have not discussed feminism, although it is a significant influence within nursing theory, as it should be in a majority female profession. Feminism is another critical line of approach in nursing, able to use the resources of the humanities to investigate and elucidate women's lives in political, social, and historical contexts.

By emphasizing certain ways of taking up the humanities and neglecting others, I have not been making judgements about legitimacy or value. By trying to establish a framework for looking at nursing and humanities at some very basic levels, I hope I have expanded the horizon of possibilities for more detailed forms of application. Likewise, as I have said at points throughout the book, nursing and humanities now makes most sense within the wider field of health humanities.

Meanwhile, there is an irony that health humanities, including nurses' contributions, has a wide horizon of possibility at a time when the humanities in their traditional home, as academic disciplines studying literature, languages, and history are threatened by shifts in higher education, as reflected in three recent books by humanities scholars (Bate, 2011; Nussbaum, 2010; Small, 2013). All three authors, two from the UK and one from the US, express similar concerns about the hegemonic force of what is seen as economically useful education over deep study and critique of human culture – STEM over humanities. One effect, which may actually have some benefit for health humanities, is that scholars in humanities disciplines are incentivized to look for alliances and collaborations with academics, practitioners, and patients in health-related areas. Bate (2011) canvassed a random sample of ten humanities scholars with a request to give a justification for the humanities to a hypothetical civil servant worrying about research funding priorities. Amongst the responses he received, one mentions using bibliotherapy in palliative care, that is, reading books to help come to terms with the emotional effects of suffering a terminal disease. Bates' unnamed interlocutor concludes, "It is not entirely frivolous to suggest that literature offers public benefits in the arena of healthcare" (Bate, 2011, p. 8). Another makes the point that "A great deal of humanities research has to do with the question of how we have come to be who we are and what we might come to be as a community in the future" (p. 8).

Some humanities scholars have critiqued their own disciplines for becoming too hermetic, too closed in upon post-modern ideology and for that reason seek out non-traditional solutions to the old two cultures divide. Edward Slingerland (2008), a scholar of ancient Chinese texts, advocates for the importance of science to the humanities, through the doorway of embodied cognition. He characterizes the university as "divided into two broad magisteria, the humanities and the natural sciences" (p. 3) where the humanities have lost their way through over-emphasizing linguistic-cultural discourses at the expense of embodied experience that keeps humanity rooted in the natural world. Another sign, perhaps of a new interest in materiality showing up in different disciplines that suggests new possibilities for cross-fertilization and collaboration.

Nursing has a distinctive standpoint – which can only be articulated with the help of humanities ways of thinking and doing derived from philosophy and history. Nursing looks out over and into the humanities with its own legacy of assumptions, social practices, histories, and beliefs. In doing so, nurses are not cut off from other health professions or from non-health professionals, but we do have things to say that no one else knows how to say. We have contributions to make to health humanities, and the wider society, in intercultural exchanges that when done well only benefit all parties.

120   *Conclusion*

References

Bate, J. (Ed.). (2011). *The public value of the humanities*. London, UK: Bloomsbury Academic.
Bleakley, A. (2015). *Medical humanities and medical education*. New York, NY: Routledge.
Jones, T., Wear, D., & Friedman, L.D. (Eds.). (2014). *Health humanities reader*. New Brunswick, NJ: Rutgers University Press.
Nussbaum, M.C. (2010). *Not for profit: Why democracy needs the humanities*. Princeton, NJ: Princeton University Press.
Risling, T. (2017). Educating the nurses of 2025: Technology trends of the next decade. *Nurse Education in Practice, 22*, 89–92.
Slingerland, E. (2008). *What science offers the humanities: Integrating body and culture*. Cambridge, UK: Cambridge University Press.
Small, H. (2013). *The value of the humanities*. Oxford, UK: Oxford University Press.

Index

Warner, J.H. 7, 8, 11
Watson, C. 85–6
Watson, J. 22, 32
Weil, S. 79–81
Whitman, W. 88
Wick, G.S. 103
Wikström, B.M. 23
Willis, D.S. 23

Wordsworth, W. 89–90
World Health Organization 40, 109

Yeats, W.B. 75, 77
Yen, W.-J. 95

Zahourek, R.P. 101
Zen Buddhism 94